THE HEALTHIEST DIABETES RECIPES

An easy way to fight diabetes by just watching your diet

OLADIMEJI MAYOWA BALOGUN

Bee research and solutions

This book is dedicated to the almighty God, the giver of knowledge and also to my deceased father, Late Mr. Nojeem Toyin Balogun.

CONTENTS

SMART EATING.

Eating right, controlling weight and getting regular exercise will help manage diabetes successfully. The following guidelines are important for diabetes control.

Whole Grains, Breads, Cereals, Rice and Pasta: These foods provide complex carbohydrates (starches), which are an excellent source of energy, and good sources of vitamins, minerals and fiber. Fiber may help lower cholesterol levels and control appetite. These foods are naturally low in fat and cholesterol. Just remember not to add extra fat.

Fruits and Vegetables: Fruits and vegetables provide vitamins and minerals, such as vitamins A and C, potassium, folate, iron and magnesium. These foods are naturally low in fat and sodium, and many are good sources of fiber.

Lean Meat, Poultry, Fish and Proteins: Meat, poultry and fish supply protein, iron, B vitamins and zinc. Other protein foods in this group are good sources of vitamins and minerals. Choose lean cuts of meat and trim visible fat. Remove skin from poultry. Eat no more than 3-4 egg yolks per week; egg whites are not limited.

Milk and Dairy: Milk products supply protein, vitamins and minerals. Dairy products are the best sources of calcium. Whole milk and high-fat cheeses are high in saturated fat and cholesterol; these fats aren't good for the heart. The best choices in this group are skim or non-fat milk, low- fat cheese and non-fat yogurt. Remember, low-fat dairy products have all the vitamins and calcium of higher fat dairy foods.

Cut the Sugar: Choose a diet low in sugar. Sugars include white sugar, brown sugar, corn syrup, honey, molasses and others. Sugars supply calories and little else. Limit foods with added sugar such as cake, cookies, candy, regular soft drinks, jams and jellies, and sugar that you add at the table.

Cut Fat: Eat fewer foods that are high in solid fats.
    Make major sources of saturated fats – such as cake, cookies,

ice cream, pizza, cheese, sausages, and hot dogs – occasional choices, not everyday choices.
Select lean cuts of meats or poultry and fat-free or low-fat milk, yogurt, and cheese.

Switch from solid fats to oils when preparing food.

Smart Cooking: Bake, roast, grill, poach, stew, steam or broil meat, fish and poultry. Use non-stick pans or cooking spray when frying foods. Trim visible fat from meat. Decrease the sugar and fat in most recipes by using vanilla, cinnamon, and nutmeg to add a sweet taste without adding sugar or calories.

10

cho ose My Plat e

tips

10 tips to a great plate

Nutrition Education Series

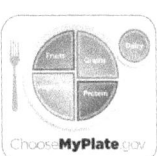

Making food choices for a healthy lifestyle can be as simple as using these 10 Tips. Use the ideas in this list to *balance your calories*, to choose foods to *eat more often*, and to cut back on foods to *eat less often*.

1BALANCE CALORIES

Find out how many calories YOU need for a day as a first step in managing your weight. Go to

www.ChooseMyPlate.gov to find your calorie level. Being physically active also helps you balance calories.

2ENJOY YOUR FOOD, BUT EAT LESS

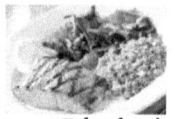

Take the time to fully enjoy
your food as you eat it. Eating
too fast or when your attention is elsewhere may lead to eating too many calories. Pay attention to hunger
and fullness cues before, during, and after meals. Use them to recognize when to eat and when you've had enough.

3AVOID OVERSIZED PORTIONS

Use a smaller plate, bowl, and glass. Portion out foods before you eat. When eating out, choose a
smaller size option, share a dish, or take home part of your meal.

4FOODS TO EAT MORE OFTEN

Eat more vegetables, fruits, whole grains, and fat-free or 1% milk and dairy products. These foods have the nutrients you need for health—including potassium, calcium, vitamin D, and fiber. Make them the basis for meals and snacks.

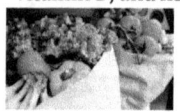

5 make half your plate fruits and vegetables

Choose red, orange, and dark-green vegetables like tomatoes, sweet potatoes, and broccoli, along with other vegetables for your meals. Add fruit to meals as part of main or side dishes or as dessert.

6SWITCH TO FAT-FREE OR LOW-FAT (1%) MILK

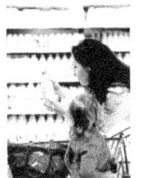

They have the same amount of calcium and other essential nutrients as whole milk, but fewer calories and less saturated fat.

7 MAKE HALF YOUR GRAINS WHOLE GRAINS

To eat more whole grains, substitute a whole-grain product for a refined product—such as eating whole-wheat bread instead of white bread or brown rice instead of white rice.

8FOODS TO EAT LESS OFTEN

Cut back on foods high in solid fats, added sugars, and salt. They include cakes, cookies, ice cream,
candies, sweetened drinks, pizza, and fatty meats like ribs, sausages, bacon, and hot dogs. Use these foods as occasional treats, not everyday foods.

9 compare sodium in foods

Use the Nutrition Facts label

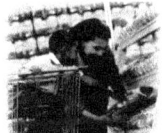

to choose lower sodium versions of foods like soup, bread, and frozen meals. Select canned foods labeled "low sodium," "reduced sodium," or "no salt added."

10 DRINK WATER INSTEAD OF SUGARY DRINKS

Cut calories by drinking water or unsweetened beverages. Soda, energy drinks, and sports drinks
are a major source of added sugar, and calories, in American diets.

DG TipSheet
No. 1

June 2011

USDA is an equal
opportunity
provider and
employer.

Center for
Nutrition

Policy and
Promotion

Go to www.ChooseMyPlate.gov for
more information.

build a health y meal

tips

10

Nutrition
Education Series

10 tips for healthy meals

A healthy meal starts with more vegetables and fruits and smaller portions of protein and grains. Think about how you can adjust the portions on your plate to get more of what you need without too many calories. And don't forget dairy —make it the beverage with your meal or add fat-free or low-fat dairy products to your plate.

1 make half your plate veggies and fruits

Vegetables and fruits are full of nutrients and may help to promote good health. Choose red, orange, and dark-
green vegetables such as tomatoes, sweet potatoes, and broccoli.

2 add lean protein

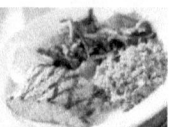

Choose protein foods, such as lean beef and pork, or chicken, turkey, beans, or tofu. Twice a week, make seafood the protein on your plate.

3INCLUDE WHOLE GRAINS

Aim to make at least half your grains whole grains. Look for the words "100% whole grain" or "100% whole

wheat" on the food label. Whole grains provide more nutrients, like fiber, than refined grains.

4 DON'T FORGET THE DAIRY

Pair your meal with a cup of fat-free or low-fat milk. They provide the same amount of calcium and other
essential nutrients as whole milk, but less fat and calories. Don't drink milk? Try soymilk (soy beverage) as your beverage or include fat-free or low-fat yogurt in your meal.

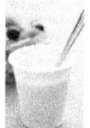

5 avoid extra fat

Using heavy gravies or sauces will add fat and calories to otherwise healthy choices. For example,
steamed broccoli is great, but avoid topping it with cheese sauce. Try other options, like a sprinkling of low-fat parmesan cheese or a squeeze of lemon.

6TAKE YOUR TIME

Savor your food. Eat slowly, enjoy the taste and textures, and pay attention to how you feel. Be mindful. Eating

very quickly may cause you to eat too much.

7 use a smaller plate

Use a smaller plate at meals to help with portion control. That way you can finish your entire plate and feel satisfied

without overeating.

8 take control of your food

Eat at home more often so you know exactly what you are eating. If you eat out, check and compare the

nutrition information. Choose healthier options such as baked instead of fried.

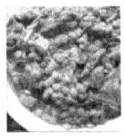

9 TRY NEW FOODS

Keep it interesting by picking out new foods you've never tried before, like
mango, lentils, or kale. You may find a new favorite! Trade fun and tasty recipes with friends or find them online.

10 satisfy your sweet tooth in a healthy way

Indulge in a naturally sweet dessert dish—fruit!
Serve a fresh fruit cocktail or a fruit parfait made with yogurt.
For a hot dessert, bake apples and top with cinnamon.

**DG TipSheet
No. 7**

June 2011

*USDA is an equal
opportunity

provider and
employer.*

Center for
Nutrition
Policy and
Promotion

Go to www.ChooseMyPlate.gov for more information.

WHAT COUNTS AS ONE SERVING?

Breads, Beans, Grains and Starchy Vegetables:

1 slice bread

½ small bagel, English muffin, pita bread, hamburger or hot dog bun

½ cup cooked cereal, pasta or rice

¾ cup dry cereal

½ cup cooked beans, lentils, peas or corn

1 small potato

Fruits:

1 small fresh fruit

½ cup fruit canned in juice or w/o sugar

½ cup fruit juice

¼ cup dried fruit

Vegetables:

1 cup raw vegetables

½ cup cooked vegetables

½ cup vegetable juice

Milk:

1 cup milk

1 cup yogurt

Meat & Others:

2-3 ounces cooked lean meat, poultry or fish
½ to ¾ cup tuna or cottage cheese
2 to 3 ounces cheese
1 egg
2 tablespoons peanut butter
½ cup cooked beans or lentils

Fats, Oils and Sweets:
Use sparingly

How many servings do you need each day?

	Women	Children,	Teen
	& some	teen girls,	boys &
	older	active	active
	adults	women,	men
		most men	

Calorie level*	about	about	about
	1,600	2,200	2,800
Bread group	6	9	11
Vegetable group	3	4	5
Fruit group	2	3	4
Milk group	**2-3	**2-3	**2-3
Meat group	2, for a	2, for a	3, for a
	total of	total of	total of
	5 ounces	6 ounces	7 ounces

*These are the calorie levels if you choose low-fat, lean foods from the 5 major food groups and use foods from the fats, oils and sweets group sparingly.

**Women who are pregnant or breastfeeding, teenagers, and young adults to age 24 need 3 servings.

2

SNACK IDEAS

Bread, toast, bagels, English muffins, bread sticks

or low-fat crackers. Air-popped popcorn or low-fat

microwaved popcorn.

Cereal snack mix. Cut down on the margarine in the recipe. Use spices such as garlic or onion powder instead of salt.

Fresh fruits, such as: berries, melon, oranges, pineapple, pears, apples, peaches, tangerines, grapes, kiwi, or exotic fruits like mangoes or papayas.

Fresh vegetables such as: broccoli, carrots, cucumbers, cauliflower, tomatoes, radishes or zucchini. Try unusual raw vegetables such as: raw sweet potatoes or jicama.

Frozen juice bars. You can make your own frozen juice bars by freezing juice in ice cube trays and inserting a popsicle stick.

Low or non-fat fruited yogurt, artificially sweetened or frozen low-fat yogurt bars.

Pretzels, rice or popcorn cakes, unsweetened cereal or

a plain tortilla. Fruit and nut breads made with whole

grains and minimal sugar and fat.

Sandwiches using lean meat, poultry, fish or low-fat cheeses. For a change, try a sandwich with all vegetables. Go light on the sandwich spreads.

Low-fat commercial snacks such as vanilla wafers, animal crackers, gingersnaps, graham crackers or fig bars.

Skim milk or hot cocoa prepared with skim milk, cocoa powder, and an artificial sweetener.

Spread ricotta cheese or low-fat cottage cheese on bread and then toast.

3

FOOD LABELS

When you have diabetes it's important to know what's in the food you eat. If you don't know, it may be difficult to achieve good blood glucose control. Food labels can help provide you with the information that you need to be able to compare foods to help you make food choices. The nutrition and ingredient information on a food label is required.

So what does the food label tell us? Let's look at it a little closer.

NUTRITION FACTS

Serving Size 1 cup (228g)
Servings Per Container 2

Amount Per Serving

Calories 90   Calories from Fat 30

	% Daily Value*
Total Fat 3g	5%
Saturated Fat 0g	0%
Cholesterol 0 mg	0%
Sodium 300 mg	13%
Total Carbohydrate 13g	4%
Dietary Fiber 3g	12%
Sugars 3g	
Protein 3g	
Vitamin A 80%	- Vitamin C 60%
Calcium 4%	- Iron 4%

* Percent Daily Values are based on a
2,000-calorie diet. Your daily values may be higher or lower depending on your calorie needs:
    Calories: 2,000 2,500

		2,000		2,500
Total Fat	Less than	65g		80g
Sat Fat	Less than	20g		25g
Cholesterol	Less than	300mg		300mg
Sodium	Less than		2400mg	2400mg
Total Carbohydrate		300g		375g
Dietary Fiber		25g		30g
Calories per gram:				
Fat 9 -	Carbohydrate 4		-	Protein 4

Serving size: Serving sizes reflect the amounts people actually eat and are stated in both household and metric measures. Serving sizes may not be the same as those used with your diabetes meal plan.

Calories from fat: Calories from fat are listed on the label to help consumers meet dietary guidelines which recommend that people get no more than 30 percent of their calories from fat.

List of nutrients: The list of nutrients include: fat, saturated fat, cholesterol, sodium, carbohydrate, and protein. Knowing the amount of these nutrients may take some of the guesswork out of meal planning.

Vitamins and Minerals: Only vitamins A and C, calcium,

and iron are required on a food label. Food companies can list other vitamins and minerals if they choose to do so.

Percent Daily Value: Shows how a food fits into the overall daily diet. You can use the Percent Daily Value information to see how an amount of a nutrient can fit into the 2,000 calorie reference diet. You may need more or less than the 2,000 calorie diet that the Percent Daily Value is based on. Your nutrient needs may be more or less than the Daily Values on the label.

4

Ingredient List: Ingredients are listed on a product by weight, from most to least. Ingredient lists don't show the exact amount of any ingredient, but they do give you an idea of the relative amount. For example, if vegetable oil is listed first, the food has more oil (fat) than any other ingredient.

Claims on the Food Label: Some food packages make nutrient claims. These claims can only be used on a label if a food meets strict government definitions. Following are some of the definitions.

LABEL CLAIM	DEFINITION*
Calorie Free:	Less than 5 calories
Low Calorie:	40 calories or less**
Light or Lite:	1/3 fewer calories or 50% less fat; if more than half the calories are from fat, fat content must be reduced by 50% or more
Light in Sodium:	50% less sodium
Fat Free:	Less than ½ gram fat
Low Fat:	3 grams or less fat**
Cholesterol Free:	Less than 2 milligrams cholesterol and 2 grams or less saturated fat**
Low Cholesterol:	20 milligrams or less cholesterol and 2 grams or less saturated fat**
Sodium Free:	Less than 5 milligrams sodium*
Very Low Sodium:	35 milligrams or less sodium**
Low Sodium:	140 milligrams or less sodium**
High Fiber:	5 grams or more fiber

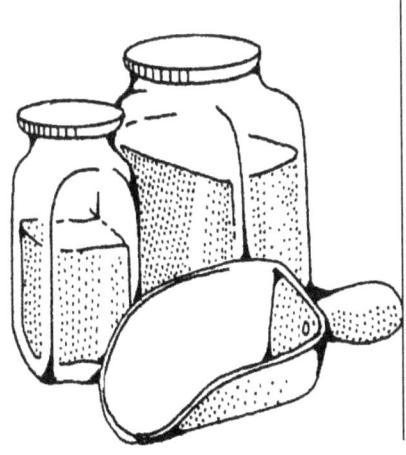

*Per Reference Amount (standard serving size).
Some claims have high nutrient levels for main dish
products and meat products, such as frozen entries
and dinners.

**Also per 50 g for products with small serving sizes
(References Amt. is 30 g or less, or 2 tbsp. or less).

5

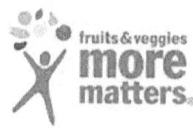

The "Fruits and Veggies—More Matters" health initiative was developed by the Produce for Better Health Foundation. The program demonstrates that eating **MORE** fruits and vegetables does matter to all of us. It's a great way to stay healthy and is a perfect fit for busy lives.

There are many potential benefits associated with eating more fruits and vegetables. Consuming fruits and vegetables is associated with a lower risk for heart disease, some cancers, type 2 diabetes, and obesity. Reducing your risk of certain chronic diseases is only the beginning. Every step taken towards eating more fruits and vegetables helps you and your family be at their best.

According to the Dietary Guidelines for Americans, fruits and vegetables are the foods that should be eaten most often. A general guideline is to make fruits and vegetables about half of what you eat, every time you eat. The current recommendation for intake of fruits and vegetables ranges from 4 to 13 servings a day or 2 to 6 ½ cups, depending on age, gender and activity level. Most adults need 7 to 13 servings a day. For most fruits and vegetables, a serving is ½ cup. A serving of dried fruit is ¼ cup and a serving of lettuce is 1 cup.

All forms of fruits and vegetables matter: fresh, frozen, canned, dried, and 100% juice. The following categories are important to eat at least several times a week because they are rich in vital nutrients:

- Dark green vegetables, such as spinach, broccoli and leaf lettuces.
- Orange vegetables, such as sweet potatoes and carrots.
- Starchy vegetables, such as potatoes and corn.
- Dry beans, such as kidney beans, black-eyed peas and black beans.

Healthy Weight Management
Research suggests that eating more fruits and vegetables is associated with better weight management. Those who consume more fruits and vegetables while cutting down on fats and added sugar manage their weight better, are less hungry, and have better intake of other nutrients such as vitamins and minerals.

Fruits and vegetables help with managing weight because they:

- Are low in calories compared to the same volume of other foods.
- Help you feel full because they have a high water and fiber content which may
help to delay feelings of hunger between eating occasions.
- Help you eat less because they require more chewing which may slow down the

pace of eating, helping to decrease intake at a meal.
- Replace foods that are high in fat and sugar.

6

Diet and Physical Activity – The Role of Fruits & Vegetables

Eating more fruits and veggies matters when it comes to maintaining a healthy weight – and it may even reduce your family's risk of many diseases. Every step towards getting more physical activity also matters in weight management and overall health. You and your family can be at your best with a balance of diet and exercise.

Research has shown that physical activity helps you lose weight and keep it off. Not only does it burn calories but there are numerous other advantages of a physically active lifestyle:

- Helps regulate the appetite.
- Helps to boost metabolism.
- Reduces stress.
- May help with insomnia.
- Is associated with a decreased risk for heart disease, type 2 diabetes, high blood

pressure, Osteoporosis.

Physical activity does not have to be about spending hours at the gym. There are many ways to become more physically active such as taking the stairs, parking at the far end of thee parking lot, walking at lunch time, getting up to change the channel, etc. The calories burned by being more active in your daily routine will add up. And don't forget recreational activities with your family and friends.

The Top 10 Reasons to Eat MORE Fruits and Vegetables are:

10. **Color & Texture**. Fruits and veggies add color, texture and appeal to your plate.
9. **Convenience**. Fruits and veggies are nutritious in any form and they're ready when you are!
8. **Fiber**. Fruits and veggies provide fiber that helps fill you up and keeps your digestive system happy.
7. **Low in Calories**. Fruits and veggies are naturally low in calories.
6. **May Reduce Disease Risk**. Eating plenty of fruits and veggies may help reduce the risk of many diseases, including heart disease, high blood pressure, and some cancers.
5. **Vitamins & Minerals**. Fruits and veggies are rich in vitamins and minerals that help you feel healthy and energized.
4. **Variety**. Fruits and veggies are available in an almost infinite variety...there's always something new to try.
3. **Quick, Natural Snack**. Fruits and veggies are nature's treat and easy to grab for a snack.
2. **Fun to Eat!** Some crunch, some squirt, some you peel...some you don't, and some grow right in your own back yard!
1. **They Taste Great!**

You can find a great deal of information at the "Fruits and Vegetables More Matters" website, www.fruitsandveggiesmorematters.org. The site provides planning, shopping and cooking tips, questions and answers, a fruit and veggie database, information about some possibly misleading thoughts about fruits and vegetables, and much, much more.

7

HEALTHY SNACKING

Snacks can be good for you! Snacks can help supply your body with nutrients that aren't in other meals and may help control blood glucose levels. Be careful that snacks are part of your overall eating plan and aren't extra "empty calorie" foods. Well-planned, nutritious snacks can prevent you from being so hungry that you eat too many empty calorie foods.

Young children may not be able to eat all the food they need at a mealtime. Children's calorie needs may be as high as some adults; however, they have smaller stomachs. Snacks should be offered according to their meal plan, which is usually 1½ or 2 hours before meals and should be given at the same time each day.

If you have Type 1 diabetes, snacks help to control changes in blood glucose levels. Snacks are planned when insulin is peaking and for physical activity. If you have Type 2 diabetes, snacks help to spread calories evenly throughout the day to help the insulin that the body makes work better and to keep blood glucose levels in better control.

The following are ideas for healthy snacking:

Prepare or buy snacks that are low in fat, sugar and salt.

Be careful of commercially made snack bars and snack foods. Many

times these foods contain as much sugar and fat as candy bars.

When you prepare snacks cut down on the amount of sugar, fat and salt used in recipes. Sugar can be reduced by ¼ to ½; fat can be reduced by ¼; salt can be cut or eliminated from most recipes (except for yeast breads).

Eat snack foods high in carbohydrates and fiber. These foods are good sources of vitamins and minerals.

Keep fresh fruits and vegetables on hand in the refrigerator. These foods make excellent quick snacks.

Look at the list of ingredients and the nutrition label on snack foods. Try to find snacks that have three or less grams of fat per serving.

Plan ahead to make sure you have appetizing snacks available.

8

Watch portion sizes. Make sure they fit into your meal plan.

If your meal plan includes snacks, don't skip them. Your blood glucose may become too low if you skip a planned snack.

Remember, when you snack, make sure the food you eat fits into your meal plan. Eating too much, or the wrong snack, can cause blood glucose levels to go up, and you may eat more calories than you want.

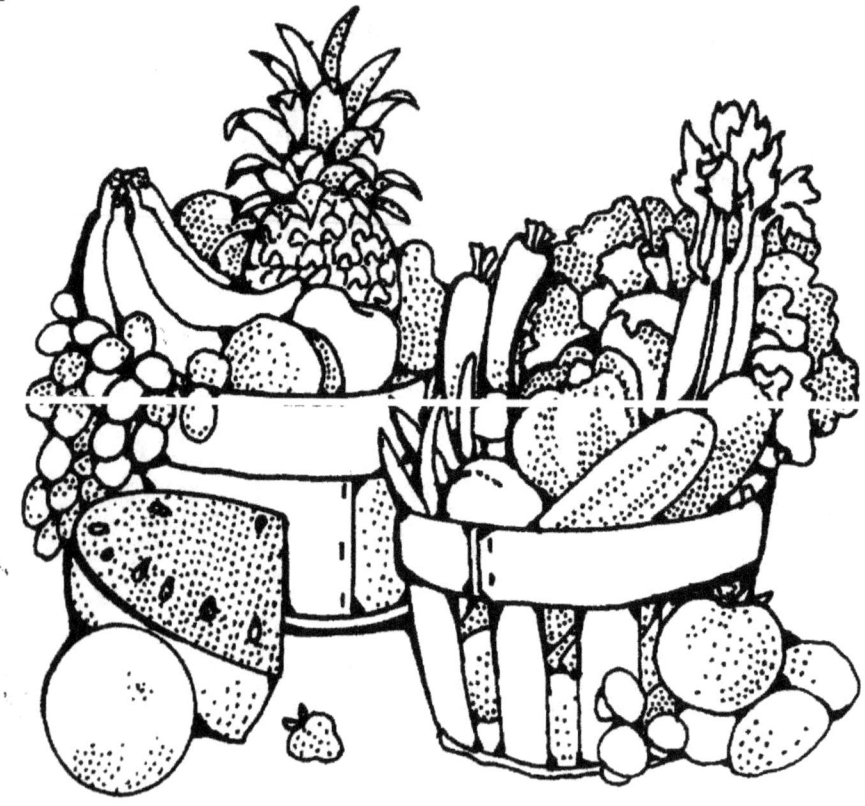

9

Recipe Ingredient Alternatives

117 cal., 5 g fat			
1 ounce cheddar cheese	1 oz. Skim mozzarella cheese		
114 cal., 9.4 g fat	80 cal., 4.5 g fat	34	4.9 g
½ cup ice cream	½ cup ice milk		
134 cal., 7 g fat	92 cal., 2.8 g fat	42	4.2 g
½ cup flavored gelatin	½ cup sugar-free gelatin		
70 cal., 0 g fat	8 cal., 0 g fat	62	0 g
4 ounces strawberries, sweetened	4 ounces strawberries, unsweetened	69	0 g
109 cal., 0 g fat	40 cal., 0 g fat		
4 ounces pineapple in syrup	4 ounces pineapple in juice		
	68 cal., 0 g fat	20	0 g
88 cal., 0 g fat			
1 ounce baking chocolate	3 Tbsp. Cocoa		
145 cal., 15 g fat	42 cal., 3 g fat	103	12 g
	10		

Recipe Ingredient Alternatives

For	Use	Calories Saved	Fat Saved
1/6 of a double crust pie	1/6 of a single crust pie		
300 cal., 18 g fat	150 cal., 9 g fat	150	9 g
6 ½ ounces tuna, oil-	6 ½ ounces tuna, water-		
packed, drained	packed, drained	123	13 g
339 cal., 14 g fat	216 cal., 1 g fat		
12 ounces	12 ounces diet		

regular soft drink	soft drink		
140 cal., 0 g fat	1-2 cal., 0 g fat	138	0 g
1 cup sugar	½ cup sugar		
720 cal., 0 g fat	360 cal., 0 g fat	360	0 g

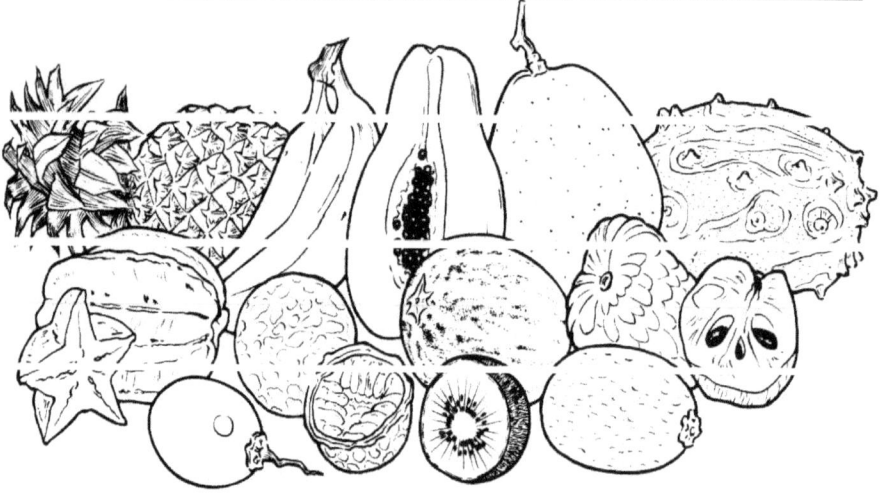

11

HEALTHY
COOKING TIPS

Sugar can be decreased in most recipes by one-fourth to one-half, and fat can be decreased by one-fourth, without affecting the quality of most foods.

When making cakes, soft-drop cookies, muffins or quick breads, use no more than two tablespoons of fat for each cup of flour. In some baked products, you can use low-fat plain yogurt, applesauce or fruit purees in place of the fat.

Use vanilla, cinnamon and nutmeg in recipes. These flavorings and spices add a sweet taste without adding sugar and calories.

Use lean cuts of meats, poultry, fish and seafood. Use lower fat cooking methods such as broiling, baking, roasting and poaching rather than frying. Also remember to trim any visible fat from meat.

Defat homemade soups, stews and meat drippings by skimming the fat off the surface, or chilling overnight to congeal the fat and remove the hardened fat from the surface.

When sautéing onion or green peppers for flavoring stews, soups and sauces, use water, stock or nonstick spray in pans.

Use non-stick pans for fat-free sautéing and frying.

Don't cook vegetables with meat. The vegetables soak

up the extra fat. Cook stuffing outside the chicken or

turkey. Stuffing soaks up extra fat.

Self-basting turkeys and butterball turkeys are higher in fat. Select a non self-basting turkey. Baste with chicken or turkey broth, apple juice, cranberry juice or sherry.

Use herbs and spices to enhance the flavor of food instead of butter.

When making salad dressings, use fruit juice to replace half of the oil in your usual salad dressing recipe. You can also add extra flavor by using herbs and spices. Try flavored vinegars in salad dressing such as: raspberry, red wine, or balsamic vinegars.

Use fruits in creative ways for a nutritious and sweet ending to a meal.

Cook to fit. If you are responsible for a special meal, plan for the number of

guests, not twice as many. Family and friends come for company and conversation, not to stuff themselves. If you prepare too much food, divvy up leftovers and share with family and friends, or be ready to freeze the leftovers.

12

COOKING TERMS

Bake: To cook in the oven with dry heat.

> **Barbecue:** To cook on a grill, over hot coals or over a fire. In some cases the food is basted with a highly seasoned sauce.

>> **Baste:** To moisten meat while roasting to keep the meat from drying out and to add flavor. Water, meat juices, broth, fruit juices and other liquids can be used.

Beat: To mix ingredients using a hand or electric mixer, spoon or wire whip.

Blend: To thoroughly mix ingredients together.

Boil: To cook foods in a bubbling liquid, usually on stove top.

Broil: To cook over or under a direct heat.

Cream: To mix sugar and fat together until creamy and soft.

> **Cut in:** To cut solid fat into flour with a mixer or fork until mixture particles are the desired size.

Fry: To cook in hot fat.

Julienne: To cut food into fine strips or shreds.

> **Marinate to** let food set in a marinade sauce long enough to enhance the flavor of the food.

Poach: To cook food slowly in a hot liquid.

Roast: To cook uncovered in an oven by dry heat, with no added liquid.

Sauté: To cook in a small amount of fat.

Steam: To cook food in steam, or over a boiling liquid, with or without pressure.

Stir-fry: To cook food quickly in a small amount of oil, over high heat.

Stir: To mix foods with a circular motion.

Whip: To beat air rapidly into a food to add volume.

13

NOTES

14

GUIDELINES FOR EATING IN RESTAURANTS

Healthy Eating Attitude – Decide ahead of time that you can go out to a restaurant and eat a healthy meal without blowing your meal plan. Too many times eating out is a signal for us to eat anything we want. Develop a positive attitude so that you can have a healthy and enjoyable meal when you dine out.

Plan Ahead – Choose a restaurant that offers healthier options. Before you arrive at the restaurant, consider what selections might be healthier.

Order for You – When you look at the menu, watch out for high fat foods, rich and creamy sauces, foods that have been fried or have extra fats. Order smaller portions. If you order a large portion, you will be more likely to eat it all.

Be Creative when Ordering – Order soup and salad or an appetizer as your entrée. Split an entrée with another person if the restaurant allows it. If you must have a dessert, split it with someone.

Make Requests – If your request is practical, many restaurants will accommodate you. Ask for a baked potato instead of fried potatoes. Many restaurants are willing to serve salad dressings, butter or margarine, gravies, sauces, sour cream or whipped cream on the side. Some restaurants have low-calorie or reduced-calorie salad dressing, or skim or low -fat milk. These items may not be on the menu but may be available if you ask.

Consider Food Preparation – Think about how the food is

prepared. Is it baked, broiled, fried, roasted, breaded, pan-fried, stir-fried, sautéed, escalloped or au gratin? Watch out for cream, butter, cheese, sour cream, sauces or gravies. Don't be afraid to ask how a food is prepared or what's in it if you aren't sure.

Know When to Stop – Many of us eat everything on our plate. Stop and leave a few bites. It's not rude to leave food or, ask for a container to take food home – you may have enough for another meal.

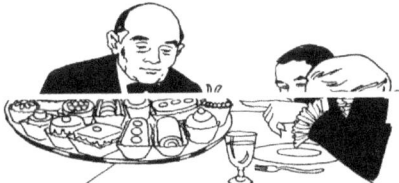 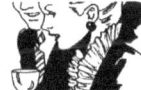

15

DINING WITH DIVERSITY

Many people enjoy the diversity of healthful, ethnic foods. Varied and interesting ingredients can be used without giving up the tastes that are part of the heritages.

French: French foods are often cooked in fat and served with rich sauces. An alternative is a bordelaise, which is a wine sauce that isn't as high in fat or cholesterol. When possible, ask for the sauce to be served on the side. Foods labeled "au gratin" often come with toppings of cheese and butter, which are very high in fat.

Italian: Bread and pastas are associated with Italian meals. Pastas are an excellent choice, as long as they aren't filled or layered with cheese or high fat meat, or have a butter or cream sauce. Good choices included marinara sauce made with tomatoes, onions and garlic; or marsala sauce, which is made with wine. Other choices include chicken and fish dishes that aren't prepared with extra fat. Dishes such as veal scallopini or Parmigiana are prepared by adding fat.

Southwest: Southwest is a blend of Mexican, American Indian, and Spanish cultures. Beans, whole grains and tortillas are staples. Be aware that lard or bacon fat is frequently used in Mexican cooking. Soft tortillas contain little fat and are good choices; however, hard taco shells are deep fried and high in fat. Lean chicken and beef that's grilled are excellent choices. Lean beef, chicken or beans (without added fat), soft burritos, enchiladas and soft tacos are good choices. Top with salsa or sauces made from low-fat sour cream or low-fat yogurt. Go lightly on regular sour cream, guacamole and grated cheese.

Oriental: Oriental foods usually contain large amounts of vegetables and rice, which are good choices. Select menu items that are boiled, steamed, sautéed, grilled or lightly stir-fried. Choose fried dishes and sweet-and-sour sauces less often.

Greek: Pita bread is very low in fat. Look for dishes prepared with small amounts of olive oil. Order dressings on the side of your Greek salad. Stick with an entrée such as kabobs that have been broiled and served with vegetables and rice. Desserts made with phyllo dough are very high in fat.

Indian: Indian food is often low in saturated fat and calories. Many of the foods are prepared with a yogurt-based curry sauce. Many salads are made of vegetables and yogurt. Vegetables and lentils are an essential part of many Indian dishes. Ghee, or clarified butter, may be used on vegetables, which may make the vegetables high in fat. Rice is often served.

Vegetarian: Vegetarian dishes are usually high in whole grains, legumes and vegetables. These foods are an important part of a healthy diet. Dishes with vegetable proteins can be low in fat, unless high-fat dairy products such as cheese, whole milk, butter and cream are used in their preparation. Nuts and seeds are also high fat foods that may be used frequently. Make sure when selecting vegetarian dishes that low-fat dairy products are used and that oils, nuts and seeds are limited in food preparation.

16

LEANER EATING AT RESTAURANTS

Appetizer: Select appetizers or hors d'oeuvres such as fresh fruit and vegetables, vegetable juices, unsweetened fruit juices, broth or tomato-based soup, bouillon, consommé, or shrimp or crab cocktails with cocktail sauce.

Beverage: Choose beverages such as: coffee, tea, skim milk, diet soft drinks or mineral waters without added sugar. (Many mineral waters have sugar or high fructose corn syrup added.)

Salad: Request vegetable or fresh fruit salads, without dressings added. Use a lemon wedge, vinegar or a known amount of dressing or dressing on the side.

Vegetables: Order raw, stewed, steamed, boiled, broiled, baked or stir-fried vegetables. Don't select vegetables that are glazed, deep-fried or with a sweet or sour sauce. If ordering a baked potato, ask for it plain or with the margarine or sour cream on the side.

Entrees: Select roasted, baked, broiled, grilled, stir-fried or blackened meat, fish, poultry or seafood. Trim off excess fat. Ask that gravy or sauces be served on the side, or not at all.

Starches: Choose mashed, baked, broiled or steamed potatoes; steamed rice; noodles; or corn on the cob.

Breads: Order breads that aren't frosted or glazed and don't have a high fat content.

Many biscuits, muffins and croissants are high in fat.

Sandwiches: Order sandwiches with smaller meat portions. Select fillings such as sliced turkey, lean ham, lean roast beef, or even a veggie filling. Hold the special sauces, mayonnaise, margarine and butter. Many special sauces are mayonnaise-based; mayonnaise is 100 percent fat. Enjoy the flavors of mustard, tomato and lettuce instead!

Desserts: Select fresh fruit, frozen non-fat yogurt, plain ice cream or sherbet, sponge cake or angel food cake.

Fats: Order margarine, butter, salad dressing, mayonnaise and sour cream on the side. Use sparingly!

If you see foods on the menu with special names, ask the server what's in the dish and how it's made. If an item isn't on the menu, ask for it. Restaurants may have skim milk, diet pop and other foods available. Choose low-fat foods the rest of the day! If you eat a high-fat meal, cut the fat later.

17

RESTAURANT FOOD PREPARATION TERMS

It is sometimes difficult to know how restaurant foods are prepared. Following is a list of some of the terms and what they mean:

a la` King: Served in a cream sauce with green peppers, pimento and mushrooms.

a la` Mode: When applied to desserts, it means with ice cream. A la Mode Boeuf means a high fat piece of beef cooked slowly in water with vegetables.

a la` Newberg: Creamed with egg yolk added, flavored with sherry.

Al dente: Pasta that is cooked to a point at which it is still fairly firm to the bite.

Almandine: Served with almonds.

Antipasto: Appetizer made up of relishes, vegetables, fish or cold cuts.

Aspic: A jellied liquid or meat juice held together with gelatin.

Au gratin: Made with crumbs, scalloped. Often refers to dishes made with cheese.

Bearnaise: A sauce of melted butter, vinegar, egg yolks, onions and spices.

Béchamel: A cream sauce made with equal parts of chicken stock and cream or milk.

Bordelaise: A brown sauce made with Bordeaux wine and various seasonings.

Cacciatore: Stewed with tomatoes, onions, garlic and other seasonings.

Coq au Vin: Sautéed in red wine and brown sauce with onions and mushrooms.

Creole: Spicy combinations of foods containing meat or vegetables with tomatoes, peppers and onions.

Curry: A highly spiced condiment from India.

Escalloped: Same as "scalloped".

Florentine: Food containing or placed upon spinach.

Fricassee: To cook by browning in a small amount of fat, then steaming or stewing.
Usually applied to veal or poultry.

Hollandaise: Sauce made of eggs, butter, lemon juice and seasonings.

18

Jambalaya: A spicy mixture of rice, tomatoes, green peppers, onions, okra and seasonings, usually cooked in oil.

Julienne: Vegetables or other foods cut into fine strips or shreds.

Kiev: Stuffed with seasoned butter and flour; often deep-fried in oil.

Kippered: Lightly salted and smoked fish.

Lyonnaise: Cooked with onions and butter.

Marinara: Tomato-based sauce with garlic, onion and other seasonings.

Mornay: A sauce with cream, grated cheese and sometimes egg yolks.

Parmigiana: Covered with breadcrumbs and Parmesan cheese, sautéed in butter, and served with a tomato sauce. Usually includes mozzarella cheese.

Remoulade: Sauce made of hard-cooked eggs, mustard, oil, vinegar and seasonings.

Sauté: To cook in a small amount of fat.

Scalloped: Food covered with a liquid or sauce, with or without breadcrumbs, then baked. The food and sauce may be mixed together or arranged in alternate layers in a baking dish.

Scallopini: Meat pounded very thin, floured, and broiled or sautéed in wine sauce.

Stir-fry: To cook quickly in oil over high heat, using light tossing and stirring motion.

Sweet-and-Sour: Sugar and vinegar added to sauces.

Thermidor: Cream sauce seasoned with wine and herbs or mustard.

Tournedos: Small round filets of beef.

Vinaigrette: Oil and vinegar combination.

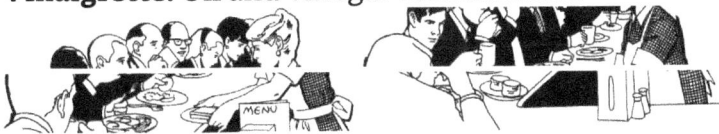

19

DINING IN THE FAST LANE

Fast food encounters are challenging. Fast food menus are loaded with high-fat foods. One of the problems with fast foods is that they tend to provide large amounts of calories, saturated fats, cholesterol and sodium. Some restaurants are responding to consumer demand with some healthier choices; however, it can be difficult to determine what the healthier choices are. Following are some points to consider when dining in a fast food establishment:

Burgers: Select the smallest meat patty. Cheese on your burger adds extra fat and calories: ¾ ounce of cheese is 83 calories and 7 grams of fat. Special sauces also add extra fat, since many are mayonnaise-based. Ketchup and mustard are relatively low in fat, but add calories.

Chicken and Fish: Chicken and fish are thought of as being lean, which they are, until they've been deep-fried. Deep-fried chicken and fish items are extremely high in fat, and may be the highest fat items on the menu. Deep- fried chicken and fish sandwiches can have 400-700 calories and contain 4 to 7 teaspoons of fat. Extra-crispy chicken soaks up even more fat and has an even higher fat and calorie content. The best choices are a grilled chicken breast or baked fish. Skip the tartar sauces (about 70 calories per tablespoon) and use cocktail sauce (15 calories per tablespoon) or lemon juice (0 calories) instead.

Sandwiches: There are many good lean meat sandwiches available such as lean roast beef, ham and cheese, and turkey. Select the junior-sized sandwiches when available. Use mustard or horseradish instead of mayonnaise -based dressings. Be careful though, as some horseradish sauces are mayonnaise-based and high in fat. If you add bacon or cheese, you are also adding fat. Hot dogs, especially the super or jumbo hot dogs, are high in fat.

Potatoes: A plain baked potato is an excellent choice. Be careful of added toppings. Toppings such as butter, margarine, sour cream, bacon, cheese or cheese sauce can add 30 to 40 or more grams of fat. Try a plain baked potato with low-fat sour cream, plain low-fat yogurt, or add chili or vegetables to keep the fat low. French fries are high in fat. A medium order of fries averages 17 grams of fat. Limit French -fries to an occasional order, split the order with someone or order a small order of fries and leave a few.

Pizza: Pizza can be a good, nutritious choice. However, pizza can be high in fat and calories. When ordering pizza, skip the fatty toppings such as extra cheese, pepperoni, sausage, olives and anchovies; select vegetable toppings instead.

20

Tacos and Burritos: Go for the soft tacos, burritos or other items that are not fried or high in fat content. Limit the amount of sour cream and guacamole. Salsa and tomatoes are low in fat, so use them as much as you want. Beans are naturally high in fiber and protein, but if they are refried they can be high in fat.

Salads and Salad Bars: Salads and salad bars can offer a healthful choice to dining out, or can be a high-fat nightmare, depending on the selections made. Go easy on dressings, bacon bits, cheese, sunflower seeds, mayonnaise- based salads such as potato salad or coleslaw, and whipped cream salads. Select salads with lots of vegetables and low-fat or reduced-fat salad dressings, or use less salad dressing.

Soups: Broth-based soups or chili can be a healthy low-fat choice when dining out. Be careful of cream soups. Cream soups may sound healthy and may even have vegetables in the soup; however, many times these soups may be made with whole milk, cream and butter.

Breakfast: Fast food breakfasts can be extremely high in fat. Eggs, bacon, sausage, biscuits, pastries and croissants are some of the high-fat breakfast choices. Instead, try bagels, English muffins or pancakes (watch how much butter and syrup you put on pancakes, or how much cream cheese you put on a bagel.) If you select a bagel, select a smaller bagel or half of a bagel. A large bagel may have twice the calories as a small bagel. Ask for low-fat cream cheese and reduced-calorie or lite syrup.

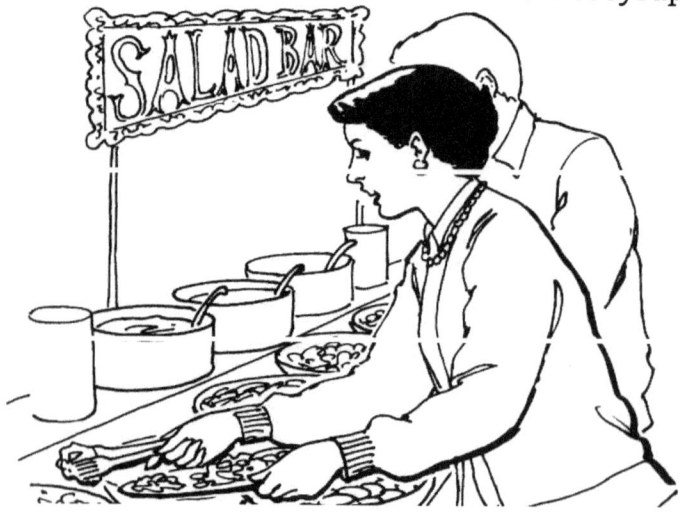

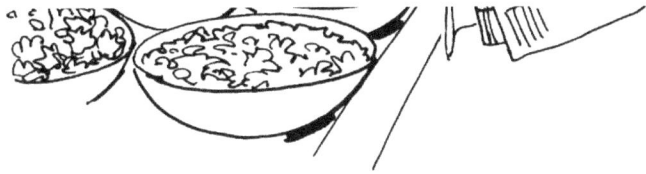

21

Take a look at the fat and calorie values for some of the popular fast foods. (Values are averages based on foods from several fast food restaurants.

	Calories	Grams of Fat	Calories From Fat	% Calories From Fat
Hamburger	275	12	108	39%
Cheeseburger, regular	295	14	126	43%
¼ Pound Cheeseburger	520	29	261	50%
Double Patty, special sauce	560	33	297	53%
Fish Sandwich, deep fried	440	26	234	53%
Chicken Sandwich, Broiled	379	18	162	43%
Chicken Sandwich, Deep Fried	490	29	261	53%
Roast Beef Sandwich	300	11	99	33%
French Fries, Medium Order	320	17	153	48%
Chicken Strips, nuggets, 6 pieces	270	15	135	50%
Pizza, cheese, 1 piece medium	253	9	81	32%
Pizza, sausage, 1 piece medium	313	15	135	43%

Chicken, fried breast	260	14	126	48%
Chicken, fried breast, extra crispy	342	20	180	53%
Chili, small	190	6	54	28%
Baked Potato, plain	300	Trace	0	0%
Baked Potato, cheese	550	24	216	39%
Taco	184	11	99	54%
Beef Burrito	402	17	153	38%
Sausage & Egg Biscuit	505	33	297	59%
English Muffin, w/ butter	170	5	45	26%

22

KITCHEN MEASUREMENTS

Teaspoons:
10 drops = dash
1/8 teaspoon = a few grains 1 teaspoon = 6 dashes
1 teaspoon = 5 milliliters
3 teaspoons = 1 tablespoon
6 teaspoons = 1 ounce

Tablespoons:
1 tablespoon = ½ fluid ounce
1 tablespoon = 15 milliliters
2 tablespoons = 1 fluid ounce
4 tablespoons = ¼ cup or 2 ounces
8 tablespoons = ½ cup or 4 ounces
16 tablespoons = 1 cup or 8 ounces

Cups:
1/8 cup = 1 ounce or 2 tablespoons 3/8 cup = 6 tablespoons
1/3 cup = 5 tablespoons + 1 teaspoon
½ cup = 8 tablespoons or 4 ounces
1 cup = ½ pint
1 cup = 240 milliliters
4 cups = 1 quart

Dry Volumes:

2 cups = 1 pint
2 pints = 1 quart

Weight:
1 ounce = 28 grams
1 pound = 454 grams

Liquid Measures:

1 ½ ounce = 1 jigger
1 tablespoon = ½ liquid ounce
1 cup = 8 ounces
1 pint = 16 ounces
1 quart = 32 ounces
1 quart = 64 tablespoons
4 quarts = 1 gallon

Equivalent Amounts:

1 pound margarine = 2 cups or 32
32 tablespoons
1 stick margarine = ½ cup
1 pound American or cheddar type cheese = 4 cups grated
1 pound cottage cheese = 2 cups
2 large eggs = ½ cup
3 medium eggs = ½ cup
1 pound all-purpose flour = 4 cups
1 pound granulated sugar = 2 cups
1 pound powdered sugar = 3½ cups
1 pound brown sugar = 2 2/3 cups
1 cup uncooked rice = 3 cups cooked
1 cup dry beans = 2½ cups cooked
1 pound macaroni = 4 cups dry or
10 cups cooked
1 medium onion = ½ cup chopped

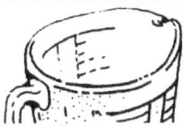
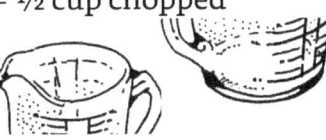
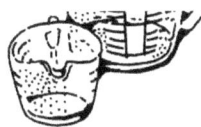

23

NOTES

24

APPETIZERS

BAKED TORTILLAS

6 corn tortillas

Cut each tortilla into six pie-shaped pieces. Place tortillas on a cookie sheet. Spread out. Bake at 400º for 10 minutes. Remove from oven and turn each one over and return for 3 to 4 minutes more. Makes 6 servings.

One serving:

Calories: 67

Carbohydrate: 14 grams

Protein: 2 grams

Fat: 1 gram

Saturated fat: trace

Exchanges: 1 carbohydrate

Cholesterol: 0 mg

Fiber: 2 grams

Sodium: 48 mg

Potassium: 46 mg

Calcium: 53 mg

BEAN DIP

4 cups cooked pinto beans   ½ teaspoon
cumin
¼ cup chopped onion   1/8
teaspoon oregano
½ teaspoon garlic powder   ¼
teaspoon salt

Mash or blend pinto beans. Mix the remaining ingredients into the beans. Refrigerate and serve. You may want to use carrot or celery sticks to scoop up the bean dip. One serving equals ¼ cup.

One serving:

Calories: 60   Cholesterol: 0
Carbohydrate: 11 grams   Fiber: 4 grams
Protein: 4 grams   Sodium: 34 mg
Fat: trace   Potassium: 206 mg
Saturated fat: trace   Calcium: 22 mg
Exchanges: 1 carbohydrate

25

Notes `

26

BEVERAGES

CRAN-RASPBERRY TEA

2 raspberry tea bags
1 ½ cups boiling water

1 cup low-calorie cranberry juice cocktail

Combine tea bags and water; steep tea in water for 5 minutes. Remove and discard tea bags; let cool. Stir in cranberry juice. Serve over ice. Makes 2 servings.

One serving:

Calories: 25

Carbohydrate: 6 grams

Protein: 0

Fat: 0

Saturated Fat: 0

Exchanges: ½ carbohydrate

Cholesterol: 0 mg

Fiber: trace

Sodium: 11 mg

Potassium: 115 mg

Calcium: 11 mg

SPECIAL TEA

4 cups water
2 whole cloves
Dash of nutmeg
peel
3 or 4 tea bags
peel

1 cinnamon stick
½ teaspoon allspice
1 long strip lemon

1 long strip orange

In a saucepan, combine all ingredients except tea bags. Simmer for 5 minutes. Add tea bags. Let steep to taste. Strain and serve. Makes 4 servings.

One serving:

Calories: 4
Carbohydrate: 1 gram
Protein: 0
Fat: 0
Saturated Fat: 0
Exchanges: Free

Cholesterol: 0 mg
Fiber: 0
Sodium: 7 mg
Potassium: 92 mg
Calcium: 2 mg

27

SIMMERED CIDER

2 quarts unsweetened apple cider   ½ teaspoon whole cloves
Sliver of lemon peel   1 stick cinnamon
½ teaspoon whole allspice

Heat all ingredients in a saucepan and let simmer for 10 minutes (or simmer in a crock-pot). Strain and serve. Makes 16 servings.

One serving:

Calories: 54

Carbohydrate: 13 grams

Protein: 0

Fat: 0

Saturated Fat: 0

Exchanges: 1 carbohydrate

Cholesterol: 0 mg

Fiber: trace

Sodium: 4 mg

Potassium: 137 mg

Calcium: 9 mg

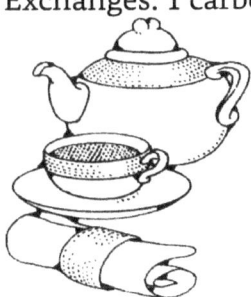

LIME COOLER

2 cans (6 oz.) frozen limeade   6 cups
chilled club soda
4 cups water   1 cup
pineapple, sliced
½ cup lemon juice   mint
springs, if desired

Mix all ingredients together. Serve chilled. Makes 20 (1/2-cup) servings.

One serving:

Calories: 37   Cholesterol: 0 mg
Carbohydrate: 10 grams   Fiber: trace
Protein: trace   Sodium: 18 mg
Fat: trace   Potassium: 27 mg
Saturated Fat: 0   Calcium: 7 mg
Exchanges: ½ carbohydrate

28

BLUEBERRY SMOOTHIE

½ cup chilled evaporated skim milk   ½ teaspoon vanilla

1 packet artificial sweetener   1cup blueberries

Put first 3 ingredients into a blender. Add blueberries a few at a time and whirl after each addition until thick and creamy. Makes one serving.

One serving:

Calories: 189
Carbohydrate: 35 grams
Protein: 12
Fat: 1 gram
Saturated Fat: trace
Exchanges: 2½ carbohydrates

Cholesterol: 5 mg
Fiber: 4 grams
Sodium: 156 mg
Potassium: 553 mg
Calcium: 379 mg

Pineapple Smoothie

2 cups pineapple juice

2/3 cup nonfat dry milk

1 teaspoon vanilla

5 or 6 crushed ice cubes

Crush ice. Combine all ingredients in a container with a tight lid. Shake until blended.

Serve at once in a glass. Makes 4 servings.

One serving:

Calories: 113
Carbohydrate: 23 grams
Protein: 4 grams
Fat: trace
Saturated Fat: trace
Exchanges: 1½ carbohydrates

Cholesterol: 2 mg
Fiber: 0
Sodium: 63 mg
Potassium: 360 mg
Calcium: 160 mg

29

CHAMPAGNE IMPOSTER

1/3 cup chilled, unsweetened apple juice
¼ teaspoon lemon
juice 1/3 cup club
soda, chilled

Add all ingredients together. Pour into a chilled champagne or wine glass. Serve immediately. Makes one serving.

One serving:

Calories: 38
Carbohydrate: 10 grams
Protein: trace
Fat: trace
Saturated Fat: trace
Exchanges: ½ carbohydrate

Cholesterol: 0 mg
Fiber: trace
Sodium: 22 mg
Potassium: 103 mg
Calcium: 9 mg

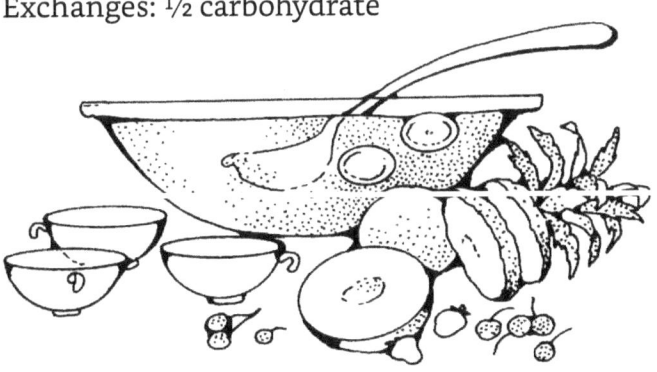

CRANBERRY PUNCH

1 quart low-calorie cranberry juice
1 quart sugar-free gingerale

Mix together shortly before serving. Makes 16 (1/2-cup) servings.

One serving:

Calories: 15

Carbohydrate: 4 grams

Protein: 0

Fat: 0

Saturated Fat: 0

Exchanges: One Serving Free

Cholesterol: 0 mg

Fiber: 0

Sodium: 15 mg

Potassium: 19 mg

Calcium: 10 mg

30

HOT SPICED TOMATO JUICE

1 46-ounce can low-sodium tomato juice

2 teaspoons Worcestershire sauce

¼ teaspoon garlic powder

¼ teaspoon sweet basil

¼ teaspoon oregano

3 drops Tabasco sauce

Put all ingredients in a large saucepan. Bring to a boil over low heat. Pour the hot mix into mugs. Makes 12 (1/2-cup) servings.

One serving:

Calories: 20

Carbohydrate: 5 grams

Protein: 1 gram

Fat: 0

Saturated Fat: 0

Exchanges: One Serving Free

Cholesterol: 0 mg

Fiber: 1 gram

Sodium: 21 mg

Potassium: 249 mg

Calcium: 12 mg

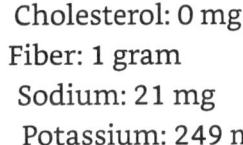

HOT COCOA

1 cup skim milk
artificial sweetener
2 teaspoons cocoa powder

1 packet

Heat skim milk. Stir in cocoa and artificial sweetener. Makes one serving.

One serving:

Calories: 101
Carbohydrate: 14 grams
Protein: 11 grams
Fat: 1 gram
mg
Saturated Fat: 1 gram
Exchanges: 1 carbohydrate

Cholesterol: 4 mg
Fiber: 1 gram
Sodium: 127 mg
Potassium: 462

Calcium: 306 mg

31

CINNAMON CAFÉ AU LAIT

1 ½ cups skim milk
1   ½ cups   strong,   brewed
vanilla-flavored coffee 1/8 teaspoon
cinnamon

Heat milk in a saucepan over low heat until very warm. Stir in hot coffee. Sprinkle with cinnamon and serve immediately. Makes 4 servings.

One serving:

Calories: 34
Carbohydrate: 5 grams
Protein: 3 grams
Fat: trace
Saturated Fat: trace
Exchanges: ½ carbohydrate

Cholesterol: 2 mg
Fiber: trace
Sodium: 49 mg
Potassium: 202 mg
Calcium: 116 mg

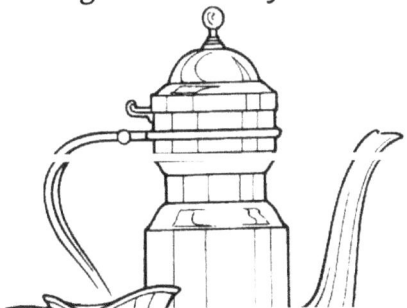

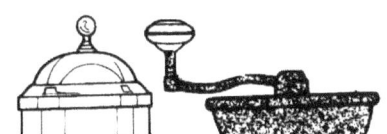

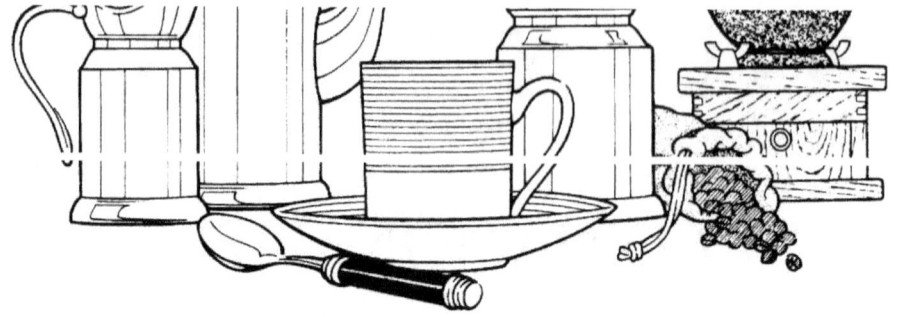

32

BREADS

BISCUITS

2 cups flour   ¼ cup
margarine
3 teaspoons baking powder   ¾ cup skim
milk
½ teaspoon salt

Mix flour, baking powder and salt into bowl. Cut in margarine
thoroughly, until mixture looks like meal. Stir in milk. Round
up dough on a lightly floured board. Knead lightly 20 -25 times.
Roll ½ inch thick. Cut with a floured biscuit cutter. Place on an
ungreased baking sheet. Bake at 400º for 10-12 minutes or until
golden brown. Makes 12 biscuits.

One biscuit:

Calories: 116   Cholesterol: 1 mg
Carbohydrate: 17 grams   Fiber: 1 gram
Protein: 3 grams   Sodium: 207 mg
Fat: 4 grams   Potassium: 50 mg
Saturated Fat: 1 gram   Calcium: 91 mg
Exchanges: 1 carbohydrate, 1 fat

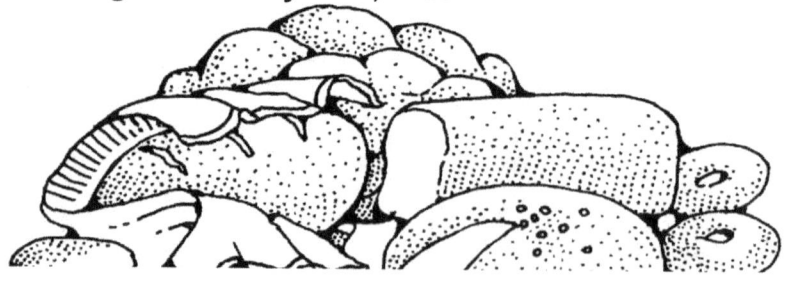

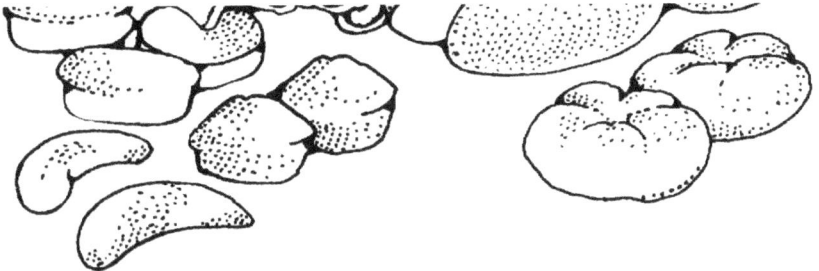

33

CINNAMON-RAISIN BISCUITS

2 cups flour
3 teaspoons baking powder
1/3 cup raisins
2 tablespoons sugar
1 teaspoon cinnamon

¾ cup skim milk
2 tablespoons cooking oil
½ cup sifted powdered sugar
1 ½ tablespoons skim milk
¼ teaspoon vanilla

Combine flour, baking powder, raisins, sugar and cinnamon. Combine milk and oil. Add to dry ingredients, stirring until dry ingredients are just moistened. Turn dough out onto work surface and kneed lightly 10 times. Roll dough to ½ inch thickness and cut into rounds with a biscuit cutter. Place on a baking sheet coated with non-stick cooking spray. Bake at 400º for 10-12 minutes or until golden. Combine powdered sugar, milk and vanilla; stir well. Drizzle over warm biscuits. Makes 18 biscuits.

One biscuit:
Calories: 93
Carbohydrate: 18 grams
Protein: 2 grams

Fat: 2 grams
Saturated Fat: trace
Exchanges: 1 carbohydrate, ½ fat

Cholesterol: 1 mg
Fiber: 1 gram
Sodium: 88 mg
Potassium: 54 mg
Calcium: 63 mg

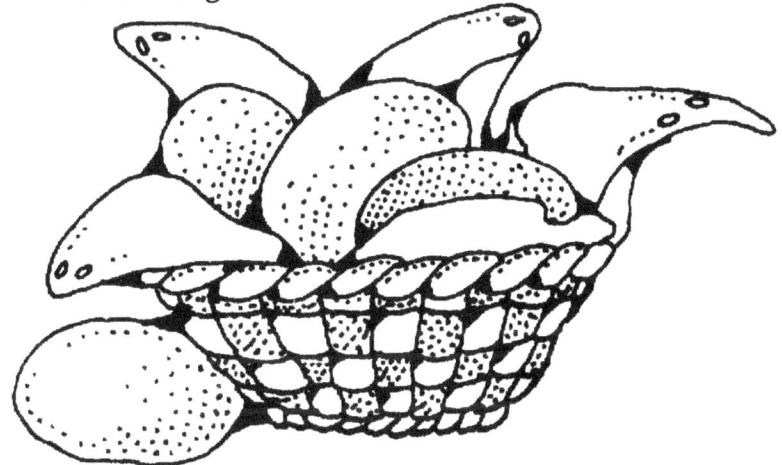

34

MUFFINS

1 egg   2 tablespoons
sugar
1 cup skim milk   3 teaspoons
baking powder
2 tablespoons salad oil   ½ teaspoon salt
2 cups flour

Oil bottom of 12 muffin cups. Beat egg; stir in milk and oil. Mix in remaining ingredients just until flour is moistened. Batter should be lumpy. Fill muffin cups 2/3 full. Bake at 400º for 20 -25 minutes, or until golden brown. Remove from pan immediately. Makes 12 muffins.

One muffin:

Calories: 117   Cholesterol: 16 mg
Carbohydrate: 19 grams   Fiber: 1 gram
Protein: 3 grams   Sodium: 226 mg
Fat: 3 grams   Potassium: 61 mg
Saturated Fat: trace   Calcium: 98 mg
Exchanges: 1 carbohydrate, ½ fat

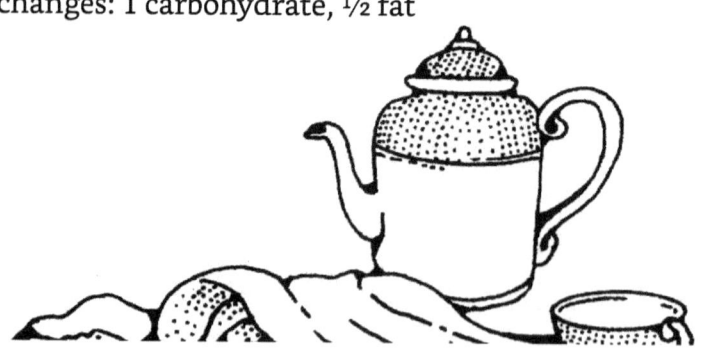

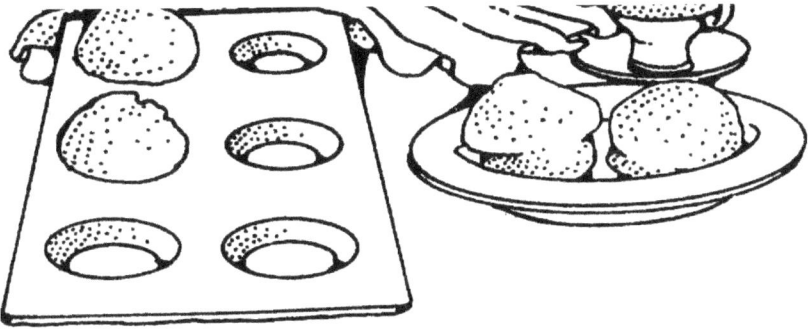

35

		Applesauce Oatmeal Muffins
1	½ cups oatmeal	1 cup applesauce
1	¼ cups flour	2/3 cup skim milk
½ teaspoon cinnamon		¼ cup sugar
1 teaspoon baking powder		2 tablespoons cooking oil
¾ teaspoon baking soda		1 egg

Combine oatmeal, flour, cinnamon, baking powder and baking soda. Add applesauce, milk, sugar, oil and egg; mix just until dry ingredients are moistened. In an oiled muffin tin, fill muffin cups almost full. Bake at 400º for 20 minutes or until deep golden brown. Serve warm. Makes 18 muffins.

One muffin:

Calories: 95
Carbohydrate: 16 grams
Protein: 3 grams
Fat: 2 grams
Saturated Fat: trace
Exchanges: 1 carbohydrate, ½ fat

Cholesterol: 11 mg
Fiber: 1 gram
Sodium: 88 mg
Potassium: 62 mg
Calcium: 33 mg

LOW-FAT DOUBLE APPLE MUFFINS

1	½ cups flour	1 egg
¼ cup sugar		¾ cup skim milk
2	½ teaspoons baking powder	¼ cup unsweetened applesauce
¼ teaspoon salt		¾ cup shredded apple, peeled or not
		peeled

In a mixing bowl, beat egg, milk and applesauce. Stir in apple. Add flour, sugar, baking power and salt all at once. Stir until just moistened. Fill oiled muffin tins ¾ full. Bake at 400º for 20-25 minutes. Makes 12 muffins.

One muffin:

Calories: 92
Carbohydrate: 19 grams
Protein: 3 grams
Fat: 1 gram
Saturated Fat: trace
Exchanges: 1 carbohydrate

Cholesterol: 16 mg
Fiber: 1 gram
Sodium: 159 mg
Potassium: 61 mg
Calcium: 80 mg

36

ENGLISH MUFFIN BREAD

2 packages yeast
baking soda
6 cups flour
1 tablespoon sugar
2 teaspoons salt

¼ teaspoon

2 cups skim milk
½ cup water
cornmeal

Combine yeast, 3 cups of the flour, sugar, salt and soda. Heat liquids until very warm (120 -130º), and add to dry ingredients. Beat well. Stir in the rest of the flour to make a stiff batter. Spoon into two 9 x 5- inch loaf pans that have been oiled and sprinkled with cornmeal. Cover and let rise 45 minutes. Bake at 400º for 25 minutes. Remove from pans immediately and cool. Makes 16 slices per loaf.

One slice:

Calories: 95
Carbohydrate: 20 grams
Protein: trace
Fat: trace
Saturated Fat: trace
Exchanges: 1 carbohydrate

Cholesterol: 0 mg
Fiber: 1 mg
Sodium: 146 mg
Potassium: 60 mg
Calcium: 25 mg

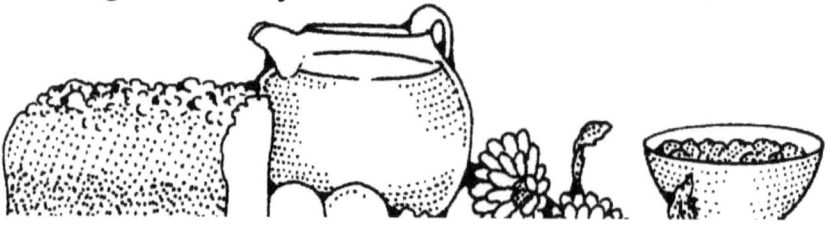

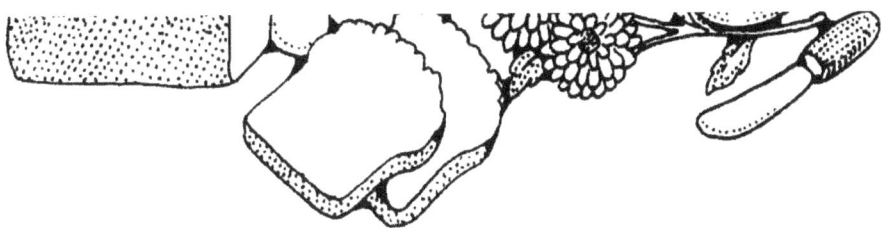

37

CRANBERRY BREAD

2 cups flour
½ cup sugar
1 ½ teaspoons baking powder
½ teaspoon baking soda
2 tablespoons margarine

1 egg, beaten
1 teaspoon grated orange peel
¾ cup unsweetened orange juice
¾ cup raisins
1 ½ cups chopped cranberries

Sift dry ingredients together. Cut in margarine until mixture is crumbly. Add egg, orange peel and orange juice all at once; stir just until the mixture is evenly moist. Fold in raisins and cranberries. Spoon into a greased 9x5x3-inch loaf pan. Bake at 350º for one hour or until a toothpick inserted in the top of the loaf comes out clean. Remove from pan. Cool on a wire rack. Makes 18 slices.

One slice:

Calories: 114
Carbohydrate: 23 grams
Protein: 2 grams
Fat: 2 grams
Saturated Fat: trace
Exchanges: 1½ carbohydrates, ½ fat

Cholesterol: 10 mg
Fiber: 1 gram
Sodium: 91 mg
Potassium: 90 mg
Calcium: 31 mg

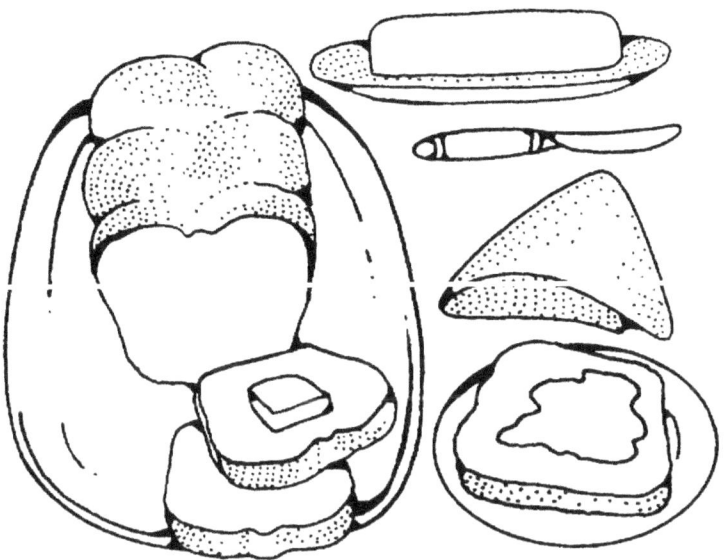

38

BOLILLOS

2 cups water

2 tablespoons sugar

2 tablespoons margarine

2 teaspoons salt

1 package yeast

6 cups flour

Heat water, sugar, margarine and salt together until slightly warm (110º). Dissolve yeast into mixture. Add 5 cups flour. Knead 10 minutes, working in last cup of flour. Let rise to double in size. Shape into 24 balls. Place on an oiled baking sheet. Let rise. Brush with a mixture of 1 teaspoon cornstarch and ½ cup water. Slash tops of balls. Bake at 375º for 30 minutes. Makes 24 bolillos.

One bolillo:

Calories: 126

Carbohydrate: 25 grams

Protein: 3 grams

Fat: 1 gram

Saturated Fat: trace

Exchanges: 1½ carbohydrates

Cholesterol: 0 mg

Fiber: 1 gram

Sodium: 188 mg

Potassium: 40 mg

Calcium: 6 mg

POPOVERS

1   egg
cooking oil
2 egg whites
1 cup skim milk

1   tablespoon

1 cup flour
¼ teaspoon salt

Beat egg and egg white together until frothy. Beat milk and oil into eggs. Slowly beat in flour and salt. Batter should be light but not foamy. Preheat oven to 400º. Generously oil popover cups; fill within ½ inch of the top. Bake immediately. Bake until very dark brown, about 35-45 minutes. When done, cut 2 small slits in the top of each popover to release steam. Bake another 5 minutes. Remove from oven. Release from cups with knife. Do not cover tops of the popovers or they will become soggy. Makes 6 popovers.

One popover:

Calories: 127
Carbohydrate: 18 grams
Protein: 4 grams
Fat: 3 grams
Saturated Fat: trace
Exchanges: 1 carbohydrate, ½ fat

Cholesterol: 32 mg
Fiber: 1 gram
Sodium: 138 mg
Potassium: 115 mg
Calcium: 58 mg

39

FRENCH TOAST
`A LA ORANGE

1　egg　　　　　　　　　　　½　teaspoon
vanilla

2 egg whites　　　　　　　1 teaspoon grated
orange peel

1/3 cup unsweetened orange juice　　　4 slices bread

Beat together the egg and egg whites. Mix eggs together with the remaining ingredients, except the bread, and pour into a pie plate. Dip bread into mixture. Heat frying pan over medium heat. Spray pan with non-stick cooking spray. Lightly brown bread on both sides. Serve warm. Makes 4 servings.

One slice:

Calories: 126

Carbohydrate: 19 grams

Protein: 6 grams

Fat: 2 grams

Saturated Fat: 1 gram

Cholesterol: 48 mg

Fiber: 1 gram

Sodium: 230 mg

Potassium: 117 mg

Calcium: 41 mg

Exchanges: 1 carbohydrate, ½ lean meat

BUTTERMILK-OATMEAL PANCAKES

1 ¼ cups skim buttermilk 2/3 cup quick cooking oats ½ teaspoon vanilla
1 tablespoon cooking oil
1 egg

1 ¼ cups flour
2 tablespoons brown sugar
½ teaspoon baking powder
¼ teaspoon salt

Combine buttermilk, oats and vanilla in a bowl; let stand 10 minutes, stirring occasionally. Stir in oil and egg. In a large bowl combine flour, brown sugar, baking soda and salt; stir well. Add oat mixture to flour mixture, stirring until smooth. Spoon about 1/3 cup batter for each pancake onto a hot non-stick griddle. Turn pancakes when tops are covered with bubbles and edges look cooked. Makes 8 pancakes.

One pancake:

Calories: 130
Carbohydrate: 24 grams
Protein: 5 grams
Fat: 2 grams
Saturated Fat: 1 gram
Exchanges: 1½ carbohydrates

Cholesterol: 25 mg
Fiber: 1 gram
Sodium: 194 mg
Potassium: 117 mg
Calcium: 56 mg

40

SALADS

APRICOT SALAD

1 16-ounce can apricots, packed in juice or water
1 small package sugar-free
lemon gelatin ¾ cup boiling
water
1 cup low-fat whipped topping
2 cups low-fat cottage cheese

Drain and save the juice from the apricots. Combine gelatin, water and ¾ cup of liquid drained from apricots. Add water to apricot juice if you don't have ¾ cup juice. Stir until all the gelatin is dissolved. Chill until mixture is beginning to set. Blend in whipped topping, apricots and cottage cheese. Place in a bowl or ring mold. Chill until firm. Makes 10 servings.

One serving:

Calories: 62
Carbohydrate: 8 grams
Protein: 7 grams
Fat: 1 gram
Saturated Fat: 1 gram
Exchanges: ½ carbohydrate, 1 very lean meat

Cholesterol: 2 mg
Fiber: 1 gram
Sodium: 270 mg
Potassium: 216 mg
Calcium: 33 mg

APPLE SALAD

4 apples, sliced in chunks
½ cup plain low-fat yogurt
pie spice
½ cup low-calorie whipped topping

½ teaspoon vanilla
¼ teaspoon apple

Toss all ingredients together. Makes 4 servings.

One serving:
Calories: 101
Carbohydrate: 24 grams
Protein: 2 grams
Fat: 2 grams
Saturated Fat: 1 gram
Exchanges: 1½ carbohydrates, ½ fat

Cholesterol: 2 mg
Fiber: 3 grams
Sodium: 32 mg
Potassium: 233 mg
Calcium: 66 mg

41

CARROT RAISIN SALAD

2 cups shredded raw carrot
3 tablespoons low-fat sour cream

¼ cup raisins

In a mixing bowl, combine all ingredients. Mix well and chill. Makes 4 servings.

One serving:

Calories: 66
Carbohydrate: 13 grams
Protein: 1 gram
Fat: 2 grams
Saturated Fat: 1 gram

Cholesterol: 4 mg
Fiber: 2 grams
Sodium: 25 mg
Potassium: 261 mg
Calcium: 31 mg

Exchanges: 1 vegetable, ½ fat, ½ carbohydrate

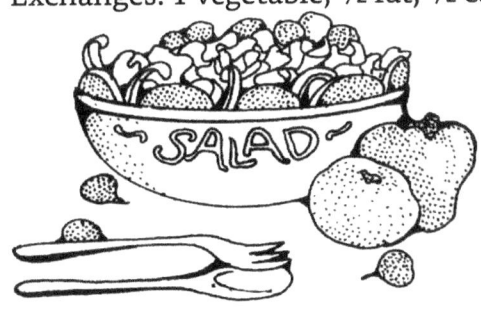

WALDORF SALAD

2 tablespoons low-fat sour cream
2 teaspoons lemon juice
walnuts, chopped
3 medium apples, peeled and diced

½ cup celery, diced
2 tablespoons

Mix sour cream and juice. Fold apples, celery and nuts into dressing. Makes 4 servings.

One serving:

Calories: 92
Carbohydrate: 16 grams
Protein: 1 gram
Fat: 4 grams
Saturated Fat: 1 gram
Exchanges: 1 carbohydrate, ½ fat

Cholesterol: 3 mg
Fiber: 2 mg
Sodium: 17 mg
Potassium: 183 mg
Calcium: 22 mg

42

CRANBERRY-CELERY MOLD

1 small package Sugar-free gelatin juice

(strawberry or cherry) ground cranberries

1 cup boiling water celery

½ cup cold water

1 tablespoon lemon

1 cup coarsely

1 cup chopped

Add boiling water to gelatin; stir until dissolved. Add cold water. Chill until partly set. Add lemon juice, chopped cranberries and celery to gelatin mixture; stir. Chill until set. Makes 6 servings.

One serving:

Calories: 17
Carbohydrate: 3 grams
Protein: 1 gram
Fat: 0
Saturated Fat: trace
Exchanges: One Serving Free

Cholesterol: 0 mg
Fiber: 1 gram
Sodium: 56 mg
Potassium: 71 mg
Calcium: 11 mg

FROZEN STRAWBERRY SALAD

8 ounces non-fat cream cheese   5 packages artificial sweetener

1 10-ounce can crushed pineapple, drained   2 bananas

1 10-ounce pkg. unsweetened strawberries   8 ounces fat-free whipped topping

Place all ingredients except for whipped topping into a blender. Blend for several seconds. Stir whipped topping into blended ingredients. Freeze in a 9-inch square pan. Makes 12 servings.

One serving:

Calories: 64

Carbohydrate: 12 grams

Protein: 4 grams

Fat: 1 gram

Saturated Fat: 1 gram

Exchanges: 1 carbohydrate

Cholesterol: 3 mg

Fiber: 1 gram

Sodium: 128 mg

Potassium: 145 mg

Calcium: 9 mg

43

MARINATED VEGETABLES

4 cups cauliflower, broken into flowerets
3 cups broccoli, broken into flowerets
1 green pepper, sliced
1 cup onions, sliced
fat-free Italian
1 cup mushrooms, sliced

1 cup carrots, sliced
1 cup celery, sliced
1 cucumber, sliced
1 8-ounce bottle

salad dressing

Mix together all ingredients. Chill and serve. Makes 24 servings.

One serving:

Calories: 26
Carbohydrate: 4 grams
Protein: 1 gram
Fat: 1 gram
Saturated Fat: trace
Exchanges: 1 vegetable

Cholesterol: 1 mg
Fiber: 1 gram
Sodium: 93 mg
Potassium: 162 mg
Calcium: 16 mg

ROMAINE FRUIT SALAD

1 tablespoon olive oil or salad oil

2 tablespoons red wine vinegar

1 tablespoon water

1/8 teaspoon salt

2 minced garlic cloves

Red onion, thinly sliced and rings separated

3 cups torn romaine lettuce

3 cups torn leaf lettuce

1 11-ounce can mandarin oranges, drained

1 cup sliced fresh strawberries

In a jar, combine the oil, vinegar, water, salt and garlic. Cover and shake until well blended. Chill until serving time. In a large bowl, combine romaine and leaf lettuce. Add mandarin oranges, strawberries and as much onion as desired. When ready to serve, pour the dressing over top of the salad; toss to coat. Makes 6 servings.

One serving:

Calories: 63

Carbohydrate: 10 grams

Protein: 1 gram

Fat: 3 grams

Saturated Fat: trace

Cholesterol: 0 mg

Fiber: 2 grams

Sodium: 53 mg

Potassium: 271 mg

Calcium: 30 mg

Exchanges: ½ fat, ½ carbohydrate, 1 vegetable

44

EASY SPRING SALAD

1 16-ounce can no-salt-added green beans chopped

1 tomato, chopped

½ cup fat-free Italian salad dressing chopped onion

¼ cup

Drain green beans; combine with onion and Italian dressing. Chill for at least an hour.

Toss chopped tomato into salad before serving. Makes 6 servings.

One serving:

Calories: 55

Cholesterol: 2 mg

Carbohydrate: 7 grams

Fiber: 1 mg

Protein: 1 gram

Sodium: 240 mg

Fat: 3 grams

Potassium: 162 mg

Saturated Fat: trace

Calcium: 22 mg

Exchanges: 1 vegetable, ½ fat

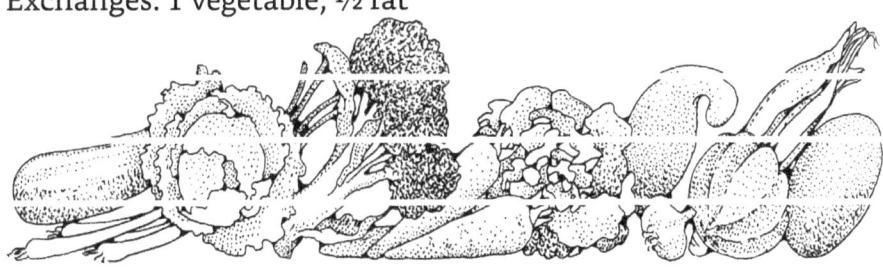

POTATO SALAD WITH DILL

6 medium potatoes   2 teaspoons Dijon-style mustard
½ cup low-fat sour cream   1 ½ teaspoons lemon juice
¼ cup fat-free mayonnaise salad dressing   ¼ teaspoon salt
½ cup chopped onion   pepper as desired
1 tablespoon fresh dill or 1 ½ teaspoons dried dill

Boil potatoes and cool. Remove skins from potatoes and cut into cubes. Add remaining ingredients; mix and refrigerate. Serve chilled. Makes 10 servings.

One serving:

Calories: 106   Cholesterol: 6 mg
Carbohydrate: 19 grams   Fiber: 2 mg
Protein: 2 grams   Sodium: 125 mg
Fat: 3 grams   Potassium: 345 mg
Saturated Fat: 1 gram   Calcium: 23 mg
Exchanges: 1 carbohydrate, ½ fat

45

BROCCOLI AND CAULIFLOWER SALAD

4 cups cauliflower, broken into flowerets

2 cups broccoli, cut into flowerets

1 cup sliced radishes

1 bunch thinly-sliced green onions

1/4 cup sliced ripe olives

8 ounces low-fat sour cream

1 tablespoon lemon juice

2 tablespoons grated Parmesan cheese

1/4 teaspoon garlic powder

1/4 teaspoon salt

1/8 teaspoon black pepper

In a large bowl combine cauliflower, broccoli, radishes, onion and olives; toss gently. In a blender combine sour cream, lemon juice, Parmesan, garlic powder, salt and pepper. Cover and blend well. Pour the dressing over the vegetables, tossing to coat well. Cover and refrigerate up to 2 hours. (You can use all broccoli or all cauliflower in this recipe as well.) Makes 10 servings.

One serving:

Calories: 62
Carbohydrate: 6 grams
Protein: 3 grams
Fat: 4 grams
Saturated Fat: 2 grams
Exchanges: 1 vegetable, 1 fat

Cholesterol: 10 mg
Fiber: 2 grams
Sodium: 138 mg
Potassium: 282 mg
Calcium: 72 mg

BROCCOLI AND BEAN SALAD

2 cups small chopped broccoli flowerets

1 minced garlic clove

3 tablespoons red wine vinegar

2 tablespoons chopped pimento

2 teaspoons olive oil

¼ cup chopped onion

¼ teaspoon black pepper

1 15-ounce can white beans, rinsed

1/8 teaspoon salt

and drained

Steam broccoli for 3 minutes. Combine all ingredients and chill. Makes 6 servings.

One serving:

Calories: 115

Cholesterol: 0 mg

Carbohydrate: 19 grams

Fiber: 5 grams

Protein: 6 grams

Sodium: 57 mg

Fat: 2 grams

Potassium: 445 mg

Saturated Fat: trace

Calcium: 69 mg

Exchanges: 1 carbohydrate, ½ fat, 1 vegetable

46

COLE SLAW

4 cups shredded cabbage
½ cup chopped green pepper
seed
¼ cup chopped onion
mustard
1/3 cup vinegar
1 tablespoon cooking oil

1 tablespoon sugar
½ teaspoon celery

¼ teaspoon dry

¼ teaspoon salt

Mix all ingredients together and chill. Makes 6 servings.

One serving:

Calories: 51
Carbohydrate: 7 grams
Protein: 1 gram
Fat: 3 grams
Saturated Fat: trace
Exchanges: 1 vegetable, ½ fat

Cholesterol: 0 mg
Fiber: 1 gram
Sodium: 98 mg
Potassium: 168 mg
Calcium: 30 mg

TABOULI SALAD

½ cup cracked wheat
3 tomatoes
juice
1 green pepper
1 medium onion
cooking oil
1 cucumber

1 cup fresh parsley
½ cup lemon

¼ teaspoon salt
2 tablespoons

Soak wheat in 2 cups cold water for one hour. Dice tomatoes, green peppers, onion and cucumber; mix together with cracked wheat. Add parsley, lemon juice, salt and oil. Chill and serve cold. Makes 8 servings.

One serving:
Calories: 106
Carbohydrate: 17 grams
Protein: 3 grams
Fat: 4 grams
Saturated Fat: trace
Exchanges: 1 carbohydrate, ½ fat

Cholesterol: 0 mg
Fiber: 3 grams
Sodium: 80 mg
Potassium: 309 mg
Calcium: 28 mg

47

TUNA AND CARROT SALAD

1 cup cooked salad macaroni
½ cup grated carrots chopped
½ cup chopped celery mayonnaise
1 (6 ½ -ounce) can water packed tuna, drained

½ cup frozen peas
1 hard boiled egg,

¼ cup fat-free

Mix all ingredients together and serve on lettuce leaves. Makes 4 servings.

One serving:

Calories: 171
Carbohydrate: 23 grams
Protein: 15
Fat: 2 grams
Saturated Fat: 1 gram

Cholesterol: 58 mg
Fiber: 3 grams
Sodium: 350 mg
Potassium: 260 mg
Calcium: 30 mg

Exchanges: 1½ carbohydrate, 2 very lean meat

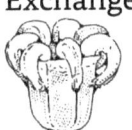 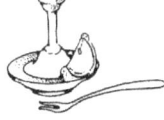

SHRIMP VEGETABLE SALSA SALAD

2 cups cooked fresh green beans

2 cups frozen corn, thawed

2 cups chopped tomato

¾ cup salsa

1 cup thinly sliced red onion

2 tablespoons tarragon-

½ pound cooked, peeled shrimp

flavored vinegar

10 sliced pitted black olives

2 teaspoons olive oil

½ teaspoon dried tarragon

Combine all ingredients and stir well. Makes 8 servings.

One serving:

Calories: 104
Carbohydrate: 16 grams
Protein: 7 grams
Fat: 2 grams
Saturated Fat: trace
Exchanges: 1 carbohydrate, ½ lean meat

Cholesterol: 42 mg
Fiber: 3 grams
Sodium: 192 mg
Potassium: 364 mg
Calcium: 38 mg

48

BROCCOLI AND SHRIMP SALAD

6 cups small broccoli flowerets
½ cup cooked and peeled shrimp ¾ cup thinly sliced radishes
1/3 cup non-fat sour cream

1/3 cup non-fat mayonnaise

1/3 cup plain non-fat yogurt 1 tablespoon lemon juice
¼ teaspoon black pepper
¼ teaspoon salt

Steam broccoli for 3 minutes. Cool. Combine all ingredients and stir well. Serve chilled. Makes 8 servings.

One serving:

Calories: 61
Carbohydrate: 7 grams
Protein: 6 grams
Fat: 2 grams
Saturated Fat: 1 gram
Exchanges: 1 vegetable, 1 lean meat

Cholesterol: 34 mg
Fiber: 2 grams
Sodium: 244 mg
Potassium: 308 mg
Calcium: 71 mg

Chicken Salad

4 cooked, skinless chicken breasts, chopped onion
(4 ounces each) slivered almonds
½ cup diced celery ranch salad dressing

2 tablespoons

1 tablespoon

¼ cup fat-free

Dice chicken into bite-sized pieces. Add celery, onion, almonds and ranch dressing.
Mix and serve cold on lettuce leaves. Makes 4 servings.

One serving:
Calories: 233
Carbohydrate: 2grams
Protein: 30 grams
Fat: 11 grams
mg
Saturated Fat: 3 grams
Exchanges: 4 lean meat

Cholesterol: 85 mg
Fiber: 1 gram
Sodium: 116 mg
Potassium: 311

Calcium: 32 mg

49

BUTTERMILK SALAD DRESSING

2 cups skim buttermilk
¼ teaspoon black pepper
parsley flakes
½ teaspoon garlic powder
minced onion

½ teaspoon salt
½ teaspoon dried

¼ cup finely

Mix all ingredients thoroughly. Chill several hours before serving. Makes 16 (2-tablespoon) servings.

One serving:

Calories: 14
Carbohydrate: 2 grams
Protein: 1 gram
Fat: trace
Saturated Fat: trace
Exchanges: 2 Tablespoons Free

Cholesterol: 1 mg
Fiber: 0 grams
Sodium: 66 mg
Potassium: 52 mg
Calcium: 36 mg

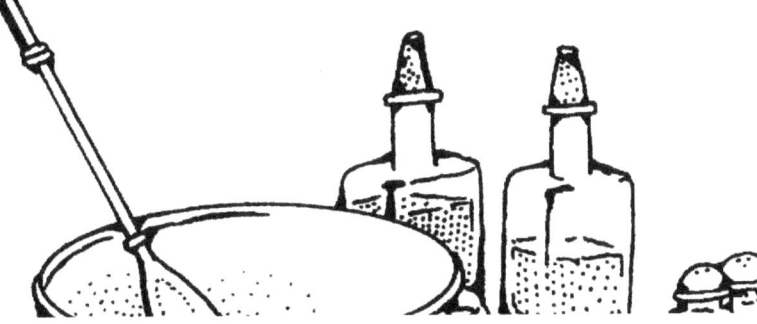

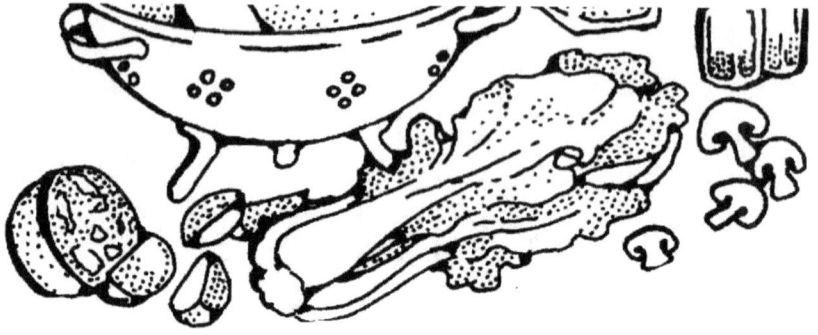

50

SOUPS

LENTIL SOUP

2 cups dried lentils
4 cups cold water
sodium tomatoes
½ teaspoon salt
¼ teaspoon pepper

1 medium onion, diced
1 28-ounce can low-

2 garlic gloves, crushed
2 bay leaves

Rinse lentils. Place all ingredients in a saucepan and bring to a boil. Cover and simmer over a low heat for 2 to 2 ½ hours, or until tender, adding water as desired. Remove bay leaves before serving. Makes 6 servings. (Freezes well.)

One serving:		
Calories: 247	Cholesterol: 0 mg	
Carbohydrate: 44 grams	Fiber: 10 grams	
Protein: 19	Sodium: 203 mg	
Fat: 1 gram	Potassium: 816 mg	
Saturated Fat: trace	Calcium: 70 mg	
Exchanges: 3 carbohydrates, 1 very lean meat		

	Minestrone	
2 minced cloves of garlic		½ cup chopped celery
¾ cup chopped onion		1 diced carrot
1 tablespoon cooking oil		5 cups low-sodium chicken broth
1 6-ounce can low-sodium tomato paste		1/3 cup uncooked salad macaroni
1 cup green cabbage,		1 tablespoon crushed

shredded		dried basil
1 cup diced zucchini		½ teaspoon oregano
1 16-ounce can garbanzo beans, drained		1/8 teaspoon black pepper

Cook garlic and onion in oil for 5 minutes. Add chicken broth and tomato paste; bring to a boil. Add remaining ingredients. Return to a boil, then reduce heat. Cover and simmer for 15-20 minutes or until the vegetables are tender and the macaroni is cooked. Serves 6.

One serving:

Calories: 222

Carbohydrate: 33 grams

Protein: 12 grams

Fat: 4 grams

Saturated Fat: 1 gram

Cholesterol: 0 mg

Fiber: 6 grams

Sodium: 100 mg

Potassium: 822 mg

Calcium: 86 mg

Exchanges: 2 carbohydrates, 1 medium-fat meat

51

POTATO SOUP

4 medium potatoes, cubed
3 stalks celery, chopped
½ cup onion, minced
1 carrot, chopped

1 ½ cups low-sodium beef or chicken broth
3 cups skim milk
4 tablespoons flour

Put all ingredient, except milk and flour, in a saucepan and simmer, covered until potatoes are tender (about 15-20 minutes). Place milk and flour in a shaker blender and shake. Add mixture to the other ingredients, stirring constantly. Simmer uncovered 5 to 10 minutes. Makes 6 servings.

One serving:

Calories: 164
Carbohydrate: 32 grams
Protein: 8 grams
Fat: 1 grams
Saturated Fat: trace
Exchanges: 2 carbohydrates

Cholesterol: 2 mg
Fiber: 2 grams
Sodium: 114 mg
Potassium: 675 mg
Calcium: 178 mg

		Tomato Rice Soup
1	½ cups low-sodium tomato juice	1 teaspoon lemon juice
1	¼ cups low-sodium beef broth	1 cup cooked rice
¼ teaspoon Worcestershire sauce		

Combine all ingredients; bring to a boil. Serve. Makes 3 servings.

One serving:

Calories: 109
Carbohydrate: 21 grams
Protein: 4 grams
Fat: 1 grams
Saturated Fat: trace
Exchanges: 1 carbohydrate, 1 vegetable

Cholesterol: 0 mg
Fiber: 1 gram
Sodium: 50 mg
Potassium: 377 mg
Calcium: 22 mg

52

TOMATO BISQUE (SERVED COLD)

3 cups fresh seeded, peeled and chopped tomatoes
1 8-counce can tomato sauce
1 ½ cups low sodium chicken broth
1 tablespoon dried basil

In a blender or a food processor, combine tomatoes, broth and tomato sauce. Cover and blend until smooth. Stir in basil. Cover and chill until serving time. Makes 6 servings.

One serving:

Calories: 41

Carbohydrate: 7 grams

Protein: 3 grams

Fat: 1 gram

Saturated Fat: trace

Exchanges: ½ carbohydrate

Cholesterol: 0 mg

Fiber: 2 grams

Sodium: 255 mg

Potassium: 400 mg

Calcium: 18 mg

SHERRIED PEA SOUP (SERVED COLD)

2 cups fresh or frozen peas

1 cup low-sodium chicken broth

sherry

pepper as desired

lemon peel for garnish

1 cup skim milk

2 tablespoons cooking

½ teaspoon grated

Combine peas, chicken broth and pepper in a saucepan. Bring to a boil; cover and cook until the peas are tender (about 5 minutes). Cool slightly and pour the peas and all of the liquid from the pan into a blender. Add the milk and sherry; blend until smooth. Pour the soup into a container; cover and refrigerate until cold. Pour the cold soup into chilled bowls and sprinkle each serving with a pinch of grated lemon peel. Makes 6 servings.

One serving:

Calories: 69

Carbohydrate: 10 grams

Protein: 5 grams

Fat: 1 grams

Saturated Fat: trace

Exchanges: 1 carbohydrate

Cholesterol: 1 mg

Fiber: 3 grams

Sodium: 80 mg

Potassium: 196 mg

Calcium: 65 mg

53

TURKEY CHILI

2 cups chopped, cooked turkey*
tomato paste

½ cup chopped onion

½ cup chopped green pepper
powder

2 cups cooked red beans
powder

1 cup water

1 6-ounce can low-sodium

1 28-ounce can tomatoes

1 tablespoon chili

½ teaspoon garlic

(*browned ground turkey may also be used)

Combine all ingredients in a large saucepan. Cover and simmer over low heat for 30-60 minutes, or until the flavors are blended. Makes 6 servings.

One serving:

Calories: 303

Carbohydrate: 27 grams

Protein: 122 grams

Fat: 1 gram

Saturated Fat: trace

Cholesterol: 40 mg

Fiber: 8 grams

Sodium: 277 mg

Potassium: 994 mg

Calcium: 98 mg

Exchanges: 2 carbohydrates, 2 very lean meat

Homestyle Chicken Noodle Soup

2 diced carrots
noodles

6 ounces uncooked

1 chopped medium onion chicken breasts,
2 chopped stalks of celery
6 cups low-sodium chicken broth

2 cooked skinless

(4 ounces each)
¼ teaspoon salt

Put carrots, onion, celery and broth into a Dutch oven. Heat to boiling. Cover and boil gently about 10 minutes. Add noodles. Cook until the noodles are tender. Add chicken and salt. Heat to boiling. Makes 6 servings.

One serving:

Calories: 213
Carbohydrate: 26 grams
Protein: 18 grams
Fat: 4 grams
Saturated Fat: 1 gram

Cholesterol: 51 mg
Fiber: 2 grams
Sodium: 208 mg
Potassium: 447 mg
Calcium: 39 mg

Exchanges: 1½ carbohydrates, 2 lean meat

54

SPICY BEAN AND VEGETABLE SOUP

4 cups tomatoes
red beans

1 cup water
pinto beans

1 6-ounce can tomato paste
garbanzo beans

1 tablespoon chili powder

½ teaspoon garlic powder
carrots

½ teaspoon cumin
celery

1 teaspoon basil
onion

½ teaspoon black pepper, if desired

2 cups cooked

2 cups cooked

2 cups cooked

2 cups frozen corn
1 cup chopped

1 cup chopped

1 cup chopped

Combine ingredients in a large soup pan. Bring to a boil. Reduce heat; cover and simmer for 20 minutes. Makes 12 servings.

One serving:

Calories: 149
Carbohydrate: 30 grams
Protein: 7 grams
Fat: 1 gram
Saturated Fat: trace
Exchanges: 2 carbohydrates

Cholesterol: 0 mg
Fiber: 7 grams
Sodium: 350 mg
Potassium: 487 mg
Calcium: 39 mg

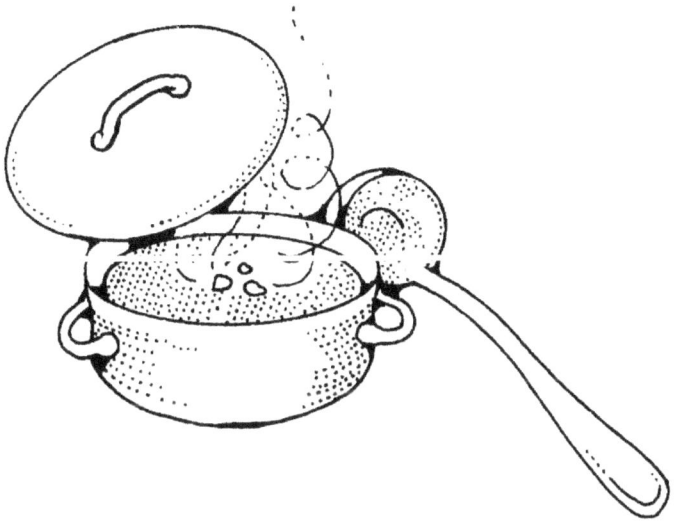

55

NOTES

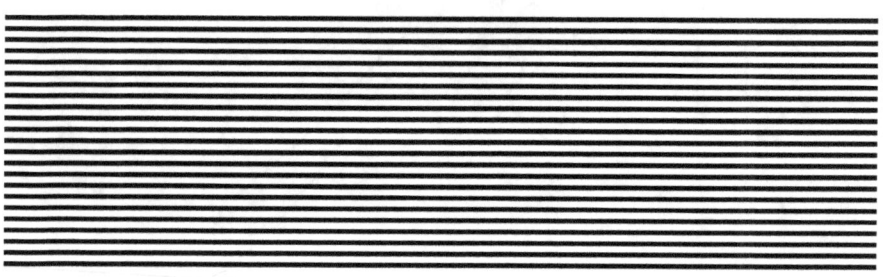

56

VEGETABLES AND SIDE DISHES

GARBANZO BEAN AND TOMATO SAUCE

2 16-ounce cans garbanzo beans, drained
sodium tomato
1 medium onion, chopped
1 tablespoon cooking oil
1 teaspoon chili powder

1 8-ounce can low-

sauce
1 teaspoon cumin

Brown onions in oil. Add spices and cook for 5 minutes. Add garbanzo beans and tomato sauce. Simmer until done. Makes 8 servings.

One serving:

Calories: 168
Carbohydrate: 27 grams
Protein: 8 grams
Fat: 4 grams
Saturated Fat: trace

Cholesterol: 0 mg
Fiber: 5 grams
Sodium: 181 mg
Potassium: 388 mg
Calcium: 52 mg

Exchanges: 1½ carbohydrates, 1 fat, 1 very lean meat

ITALIAN-MEXICAN VEGETABLE BAKE

1	10-ounce package frozen Italian beans	16-ounce can low-sodium corn
1	½ cups cooked, drained garbanzo beans	1 16-ounce can low-sodium
1	4-ounce can green chilies, drained	tomatoes
	dash of hot sauce	1 cup (4 oz.) shredded Monterey Jack
		Cheese

In a casserole dish, mix all ingredients except cheese. Top mixture with cheese.

Bake at 350º for 30 minutes. Makes 10 servings.

One serving:

Calories: 136
Carbohydrate: 20 grams
Protein: 7 grams
Fat: 5 grams
Saturated Fat: 2 grams

Cholesterol: 10 mg
Fiber: 4 grams
Sodium: 209 mg
Potassium: 323 mg
Calcium: 125 mg

Exchanges: 1 carbohydrate, ½ fat, ½ medium-fat meat

57

PARMESAN BASIL TOMATOES

2 cups fresh or low-sodium canned tomatoes, diced   1 teaspoon basil

¼ teaspoon garlic powder   1/8 teaspoon black pepper

2 tablespoons Parmesan cheese

Mix all ingredients except the Parmesan cheese in a sauce pan; heat. Serve with Parmesan cheese sprinkled on top. Makes 4 servings.

One serving:

Calories: 40

Carbohydrate: 6 grams

Protein: 3 grams

Fat: 1 gram

Saturated Fat: 1 gram

Cholesterol: 2 mg

Fiber: 2 grams

Sodium: 74 mg

Potassium: 282 mg

Calcium: 85 mg

Exchanges: 1 vegetable, 1 very lean meat

SCALLOPED CORN

2 16-ounce cans whole kernel, no-added-salt corn
2 tablespoons flour
1 tablespoon sugar
¼ cup milk

1 egg, beaten
2 egg whites
1 tablespoon dried minced onion ½ green pepper, chopped
4 oz. shredded cheddar cheese

Drain corn. Place corn, flour and sugar in an oiled baking dish and mix. Add milk, egg, egg whites, onion and green pepper. Mix well. Sprinkle cheddar cheese on top. Bake in oven at 400º for 35-40 minutes, or until set. Makes 8 servings.

Note: For a more festive flavor, substitute a 4-ounce can of green chilies for the green peppers

One serving:

Calories: 141
Carbohydrate: 24 grams
Protein: 6 grams
chiles add   mg)
Fat: 4 grams
Saturated Fat: 2 grams
Exchanges: 1½ carbohydrates, ½ fat

Cholesterol: 31 mg
Fiber: 2 grams
 Sodium: 72 mg (green

 Potassium: 246 mg
Calcium: 19 mg

GREEN BEAN CASSEROLE

1 teaspoon cooking oil
¼ cup chopped onion
2 tablespoons flour
1 cup skim milk
1/3 cup shredded, reduced-fat Swiss cheese
½ cup low-fat sour cream

1 teaspoon sugar
¼ teaspoon salt
1 16-ounce package frozen green beans, thawed and drained
1 cup herb-seasoned stuffing mix
1 teaspoon margarine, melted

In a medium saucepan, sauté onion in cooking oil. Add flour and cook 1 minute, stirring constantly. Gradually add the milk, stirring until blended. Stir in cheese, sour cream, sugar and salt. Cook for 5 minutes or until thickened and bubbly, stirring constantly. Put green beans in a baking dish; pour sauce over the top. In another bowl, pour the melted margarine over the stuffing mix; stir well and sprinkle over green bean mixture. Bake at 350º for 20-25 minutes or until heated through. Makes 8 servings.

One serving:

Calories: 106
Carbohydrate: 11 grams
Protein: 5 grams
Fat: 5 grams

Cholesterol: 8 mg
Fiber: 2 grams
Sodium: 186 mg
Potassium: 160 mg

Saturated Fat: 2 grams   Calcium: 138 mg
Exchanges: 1½ carbohydrates, 1 fat, 1 vegetable

TWICE BAKED YAMS

2 medium yams
2 tablespoons skim milk

Wrap yams in foil. Bake at 350º for one hour or until tender. Split yams in half, lengthwise. Scoop out contents and whip with milk. Spoon back into potato shells and heat thoroughly in oven. Makes 4 servings.

One serving:

Calories: 62

Carbohydrate: 14 grams

Protein: 1 gram

Fat: trace

Saturated Fat: trace

Exchanges: 1 carbohydrate

Cholesterol: trace

Fiber: 2 grams

Sodium: 10 mg

Potassium: 213 mg

Calcium: 26 mg

59

GRILLED VEGETABLES AND POTATOES

2 large potatoes, sliced, washed and unpeeled
2 sliced carrots
1 sliced onion

Spray a large piece of aluminum foil with non -stick cooking spray. Place potatoes, carrots and onions on aluminum foil. Sprinkle with one tablespoon water. Fold foil around vegetables and seal. Place on a slow charcoal grill or a gas grill on low for about 30 minutes or until vegetables are tender. Makes 4 servings.

One serving:

Calories: 99
Carbohydrate: 23 grams
Protein: 2 grams
Fat: trace
Saturated Fat: trace
Exchanges: 1 carbohydrate, 1 vegetable

Cholesterol: 0 mg
Fiber: 3 grams
Sodium: 17 mg
Potassium: 465 mg
Calcium: 19 mg

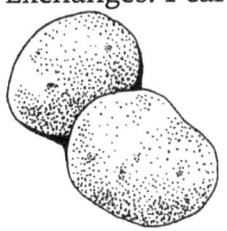

MICROWAVED CHEESE POTATO FRIES

4 scrubbed potatoes
¼ teaspoon garlic powder
½ cup shredded, low-fat mozzarella cheese

Cut potatoes into strips. Put potatoes in a large baking dish, single layered. Sprinkle with garlic powder and cheese. Cover and microwave on full power for about 12 minutes or until potatoes are tender. Makes 8 servings.

One serving:

Calories: 93

Carbohydrate: 17 grams

Protein: 4 grams

Fat: 1 gram

Saturated Fat: 1 gram

Exchanges: 1 carbohydrate

Cholesterol: 4 mg

Fiber: 1 gram

Sodium: 41 mg

Potassium: 312 mg

Calcium: 56 mg

60

GREEN BEAN AND RICE CASSEROLE

½ cup chopped onion

2 teaspoons cooking oil

½ cup uncooked rice

1 16-ounce can low-sodium green beans

1 16-ounce can tomatoes

1/3 cup water

Sauté the onions in cooking oil until brown. Combine all ingredients and place in a baking dish. Cook, covered, for 30 minutes. Makes 4 servings.

One serving:

Calories: 126

Carbohydrate: 23 grams

Protein: 4 grams

Fat: 3 grams

Saturated Fat: trace

Cholesterol: 0 mg

Fiber: 3 grams

Sodium: 200 mg

Potassium: 432 mg

Calcium: 69 mg

Exchanges: 1 carbohydrate, ½ fat, 1 vegetable

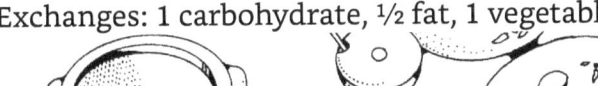

SWEET AND SOUR CABBAGE

6 cups chopped cabbage

1/8 teaspoon black pepper

1 cup chopped onion

1 minced garlic clove

2 teaspoons olive oil

3 tablespoons wine vinegar

1/8 teaspoon salt

1 tablespoon honey

Combine all ingredients and place in a baking dish. Cover and bake at 400º for 30 minutes or until tender. Stir and serve. Makes 4 servings.

One serving:

Calories: 80

Cholesterol: 0 mg

Carbohydrate: 14 grams

Fiber: 3 grams

Protein: 2 grams

Sodium: 87 mg

Fat: 3 grams

Potassium: 339 mg

Saturated Fat: trace

Calcium: 60 mg

Exchanges: 1 carbohydrate, ½ fat

61

RICE OLE`

1 cup chopped onion powder
1 cup chopped green pepper
1 tablespoon vegetable oil tomatoes
2 teaspoons chili powder

½ teaspoon garlic
¼ teaspoon salt
1 16-ounce can
3 cups cooked rice

Sauté onions and green pepper in oil until vegetables are tender but not brown. Add seasonings, salt, tomatoes and rice. Simmer and stir until flavors are blended and liquid is absorbed (about 10 minutes). Makes 10 servings.

One serving:

Calories: 113
Carbohydrate: 22 grams
Protein: 3 grams
Fat: 2 grams
Saturated Fat: trace

Cholesterol: 0 mg
Fiber: 1 gram
Sodium: 138 mg
Potassium: 181 mg
Calcium: 24 mg

Exchanges: 1 carbohydrate, ½ fat, 1 vegetable

SPANISH RICE

1 tablespoon cooking oil
½ cup chopped onion
rice
¼ cup celery, chopped
tomatoes
1 cup water
lean ground beef, cooked,

¼ teaspoon salt
¾ cup uncooked

2 cups diced

½ pound extra

with fat drained

In a large skillet, brown onions and celery in cooking oil. Add water, salt, rice and tomatoes. Simmer until rice is tender (about 15 minutes), stirring occasionally. Add meat and cook slowly, stirring, until heated through (about 5-10 minutes). Makes 6 servings.

One serving:

Calories: 201
Carbohydrate: 23 grams
Protein: 11 grams
Fat: 7 grams
Saturated Fat: 2 grams

Cholesterol: 28 mg
Fiber: 1 gram
Sodium: 249 mg
Potassium: 343 mg
Calcium: 35 mg

Exchanges: 1 carbohydrate, ½ fat, 1 vegetable, 1 medium-fat meat

FESTIVE RICE

½ cup chopped onion
½ cup chopped celery
broccoli
½ cup chopped green pepper
1 tablespoon margarine

2 cups cooked rice
1 cup cooked

¼ teaspoon salt

Sauté onion, celery and green pepper in margarine. Add rice, broccoli and salt. Stir well and cook until mixture is heated through. Makes 6 servings.

One serving:

Calories: 122
Carbohydrate: 23 grams
Protein: 3 grams
Fat: 2 grams
Saturated Fat: trace

Cholesterol: 0 mg
Fiber: 2 grams
Sodium: 122 mg
Potassium: 165 mg
Calcium: 27 mg

Exchanges: 1 carbohydrate, ½ fat, 1 vegetable

RED BEANS AND RICE

½ cup chopped onion

red beans

½ cup chopped celery

1 minced garlic clove pepper

1 tablespoon margarine

2 cups pre-cooked

2 cups cooked rice

1/8 teaspoon

Cook onion, celery and garlic in margarine until tender. Add remaining ingredients.

Simmer together for 5 minutes to blend flavors. Makes 6 servings.

One serving:

Calories: 151

Carbohydrate: 26 grams

Protein: 6 grams

Fat: 3 grams

Saturated Fat: trace

Exchanges: 1½ carbohydrate, ½ fat

Cholesterol: 0 mg

Fiber: 6 grams

Sodium: 319 mg

Potassium: 293 mg

Calcium: 34 mg

63

WILD RICE CASSEROLE

1 cup uncooked wild rice
3 cups low-sodium chicken broth
¼ cup chopped onion
½ cup chopped mushrooms

¼ teaspoon pepper
¼ teaspoon salt
¼ teaspoon sage

Using non-stick cooking spray, coat the inside of a saucepan and sauté onions and mushrooms. Rinse wild rice in water before using. Add wild rice, broth, pepper, salt and sage to the onions and mushrooms. Bring to a boil. Simmer for 40-50 minutes, stirring occasionally. Makes 6 servings.

One serving:

Calories: 131
Carbohydrate: 24 grams
Protein: 7 grams
Fat: 1 gram
Saturated Fat: trace
Exchanges: 1½ carbohydrates

Cholesterol: 0 mg
Fiber: 2 grams
Sodium: 128 mg
Potassium: 244 mg
Calcium: 11 mg

BREAD STUFFING

1 low-sodium chicken bouillon cube ¾ cup boiling water
¼ cup chopped onion ¼ cup diced celery

4 cups (6 slices) dry bread cubes
½ teaspoon poultry seasoning
½ teaspoon dried sage, crushed 1/8 teaspoon pepper, if desired

Dissolve bouillon cube in boiling water. Add chopped onion and celery to bouillon and simmer 5 minutes. Combine bread cubes and seasonings. Pour bouillon mixture over bread and toss gently until moistened. Use as a stuffing or bake in an 8x8-inch dish at 325º for 25-30 minutes. Makes 6 servings.

One serving:

Calories: 101
Carbohydrate: 18 grams
Protein: 4 grams
Fat: 2 grams
Saturated Fat: trace
Exchanges: 1 carbohydrate

Cholesterol: 1 mg
Fiber: 1 gram
Sodium: 180 mg
Potassium: 100 mg
Calcium: 38 mg

64

NORTHLANDS WILD RICE CASSEROLE

1 cup uncooked wild rice
2 cups low-sodium chicken broth

1 tablespoon margarine
1 cup sliced fresh mushrooms ¾ cup sliced celery
¾ cup julienned carrots

1/3 cup sliced green onion
¼ cup chopped sweet red pepper
½ teaspoon dried thyme
¼ teaspoon salt
¼ teaspoon black pepper

Rinse wild rice under running water for one minute; drain and set aside. In a medium saucepan, combine the chicken broth and wild rice. Bring to a boil. Reduce heat; cover and simmer for 30 minutes. In a large skillet, melt margarine and add mushrooms, carrots and celery. Cook and stir for 5 minutes. Stir in green onion, sweet red pepper, thyme, salt and pepper. Stir the rice into the vegetable mixture. Put the mixture into a casserole dish. Bake, covered, at 325º for about 45 minutes, or until the rice is done. Makes 8 servings.

One serving:

Calories: 117
Carbohydrate: 20 grams
Protein: 5 grams
Fat: 2 grams

Cholesterol: 0 mg
Fiber: 2 grams
Sodium: 120 mg
Potassium: 265 mg

Saturated Fat: trace   Calcium: 20 mg
Exchanges: 1 carbohydrate, ½ fat, 1 vegetable

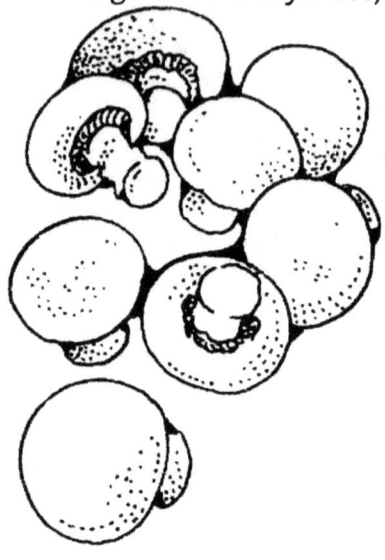

65

NOTES

66

POULTRY, FISH AND MAIN DISHES

CHICKEN CILANTRO

1 small onion, chopped
1 garlic clove, finely chopped
1 tablespoon margarine
4 small chicken breasts, boned, skinned, cut into
pieces (4 ounces each) 1/8 teaspoon salt
¼ teaspoon black pepper, if desired
2 tablespoons cilantro, snipped

In a skillet, cook onions and garlic in margarine until onion is tender. Add chicken, salt and pepper. Cook and stir over medium-high heat about 5- 10 minutes. Stir in cilantro. Garnish with a lemon wedge if desired. Makes 4 servings.

One serving:

Calories: 180
Carbohydrate: 3 grams
Protein: 27 grams
Fat: 6 grams
Saturated Fat: 1 gram
Exchanges: 3 ½ lean meat, 1 vegetable

Cholesterol: 73 mg
Fiber: 1 gram
Sodium: 159 mg
Potassium: 272 mg
Calcium: 22 mg

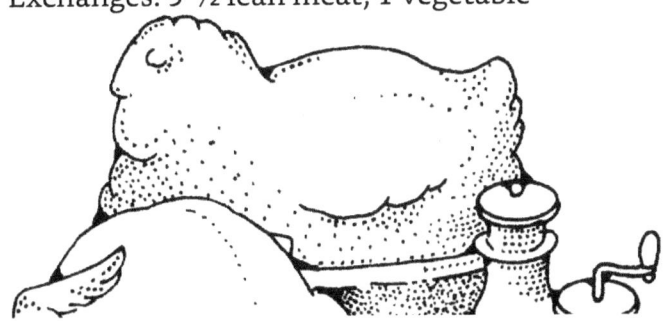

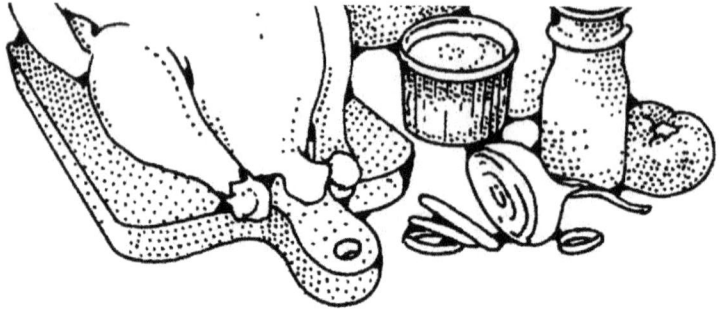

67

CHICKEN ENCHILADAS

½ cup chopped onion

1 teaspoon cooking oil

4 ounces reduced-fat cream cheese

1 tablespoon water

1 teaspoon ground cumin

1/8 teaspoon black pepper

1/8 teaspoon salt

4 cups chopped, cooked, skinless chicken breast, (4 ounces each)

12 8-inch flour tortillas

1 10 ¾-ounce can reduced-fat, reduced-sodium condensed cream of chicken soup

8 ounces low-fat sour cream

1 cup skim milk

1 4-ounce can chopped green chilies

½ cup shredded cheddar cheese

In a small skillet, sauté onion in oil. In a mixing bowl, stir together cream cheese, water, cumin, black pepper and salt. Stir cooked onion and chicken into cream cheese mixture. Wrap tortillas in foil and heat in a 350º oven for 10 minutes, or until softened. Spoon about ¼ cup of the chicken mixture onto each tortilla. Roll up the tortillas and place seam side down on a baking dish that has been sprayed with non-stick cooking spray. To make sauce, combine soup, sour cream, milk and green chilies; pour over enchiladas. Bake, covered at 350º for 40 minutes or until heated through. Sprinkle with cheddar cheese. Bake, uncovered, for 5 minutes or until cheese is melted. Makes 12 enchiladas.

One enchilada:

Calories: 288

Carbohydrate: 25 grams

Protein: 21 grams

Fat: 11 grams

Saturated Fat: 2 grams

Cholesterol: 58 mg

Fiber: 1 gram

Sodium: 414 mg

Potassium: 305 mg

Calcium: 153 mg

Exchanges: 1½ carbohydrates, 2 medium-fat meat

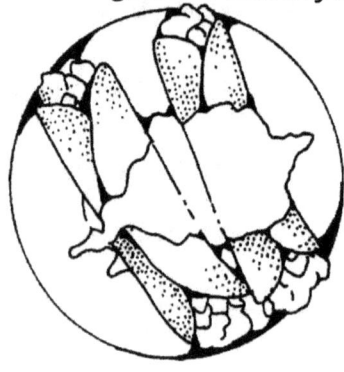

68

RICE MEAT BALLS

1 cup instant rice
1 pound extra-lean ground beef
marjoram
1 egg, slightly beaten
¼ cup grated onion
sodium tomato juice
¼ cup grated onion

¼ teaspoon salt
1/8 teaspoon

dash of pepper
2 ½ cups low-

Mix all ingredients together except 2 cups of the tomato juice. Form into meatballs. Place meatballs into a skillet. Brown meatballs and drain off any fat. Pour remaining tomato juice over meatballs. Bring to a boil; reduce to medium heat; cover and cook for 15 minutes. Makes 6 servings.

One serving:

Calories: 241
Carbohydrate: 18 grams
Protein: 19 grams
Fat: 10 grams
Saturated Fat: 4 grams
Exchanges: 2 medium-fat meat, 1 carbohydrate

Cholesterol: 87 mg
Fiber: 1 grams
Sodium: 152 mg
Potassium: 456 mg
Calcium: 22 mg

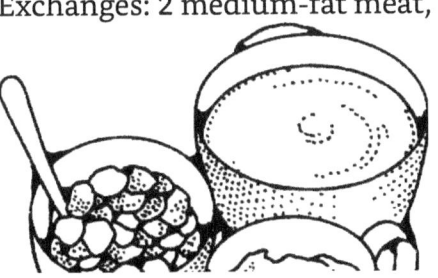
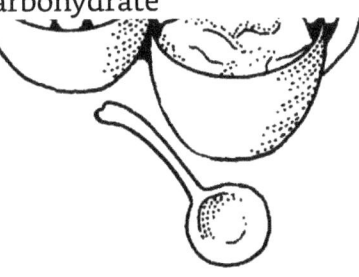

69

SWEDISH CABBAGE ROLLS

1 egg
1 pound extra-lean ground beef
1/4 teaspoon salt
3/4 cup cooked rice
pepper (as desired)
6 large cabbage leaves
1 teaspoon Worcestershire sauce
1 cup low-sodium tomato juice
1/4 cup chopped onion
1 tablespoon lemon juice
1/3 cup skim milk
1 tablespoon brown sugar

Combine egg, salt, pepper, Worcestershire sauce, onion and milk. Mix well. Add ground beef and cooked rice; beat together with a fork. Immerse cabbage leaves in boiling water for 3 minutes or just until limp. Drain. Place ½ cup meat mixture on each cabbage leaf; fold in sides and roll ends over meat. Place rolls in a baking dish. Blend tomato juice, brown sugar and lemon juice. Pour over cabbage rolls. Bake at 350º for 1 hour. Makes 6 servings.

One cabbage roll:

Calories: 214
Cholesterol: 88 mg
Carbohydrate: 12 grams
Fiber: 2 grams
Protein: 19 grams
Sodium: 171 mg
Fat: 10 grams
Potassium: 415 mg
Saturated Fat: 4 grams
Calcium: 36 mg

Exchanges: 2 medium-fat meat, 1 carbohydrate

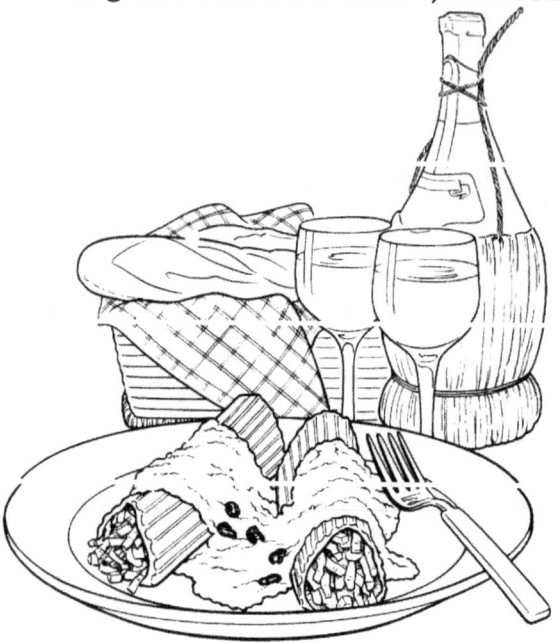

70

BEEF BURGUNDY

1 pound lean beef, cubed
¼ cup flour
1/8 teaspoon pepper
2 tablespoons cooking oil
½ cup chopped onion
1 garlic clove
¼ teaspoon thyme
¼ teaspoon basil
¼ teaspoon oregano

1/8 teaspoon rosemary
1 tablespoon parsley
½ cup dry red cooking wine
1 cup water
2 cups chopped fresh tomatoes
2 cups diced raw carrots
2 cups sliced raw mushrooms
3 cups diced potatoes

Coat beef with flour and pepper. Brown meat in oil. Add onion and garlic, then cook until tender. Pour off fat. Add spices, wine and water. Cover and simmer for 30 minutes, stirring occasionally, adding more water if necessary. Add tomatoes, carrots, mushrooms and potatoes; simmer one more hour. Makes 8 servings.

One serving:

Calories: 197
Carbohydrate: 19 grams
Protein: 15 grams
Fat: 6 grams
Saturated Fat: 2 grams

Cholesterol: 38 mg
Fiber: 3 grams
Sodium: 43 mg
Potassium: 635 mg
Calcium: 25 mg

Exchanges: 1 vegetable, 1½ lean meat, 1 carbohydrate

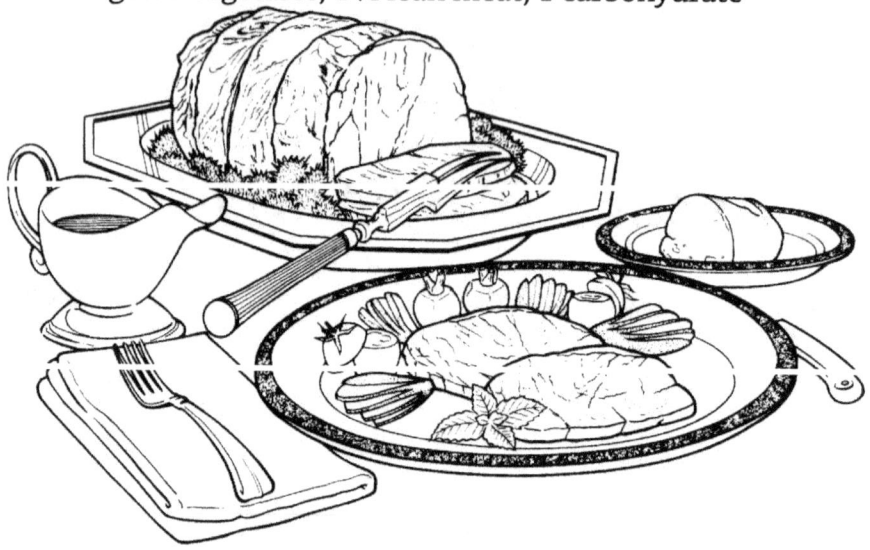

71

FRUITY HAM SLICES

1 pound low-sodium, extra lean ham slices (8 slices)
2 bananas
½ cup crushed pineapple in juice
1 cup unsweetened pineapple juice
2 teaspoons cornstarch
½ teaspoon cinnamon
1/8 teaspoon ground cloves

Place ham slices in a baking dish. Peel bananas and cut into quarters, lengthwise. Place ¼ banana and 1 tablespoon crushed pineapple on each ham slice. To make sauce, pour pineapple juice in a saucepan. Add cornstarch, cinnamon and cloves.
Cook over medium heat until juice is clear and slightly thickened. Pour sauce over top of ham. Bake 20 minutes at 350º. Makes 8 servings.

One serving:

Calories: 142
Carbohydrate: 15 grams
Protein: 12 grams
Fat: 3 grams
Saturated Fat: 1 gram
Exchanges: 1 carbohydrate, 2 very-lean meat

Cholesterol: 30mg
Fiber: 2 grams
Sodium: 550 mg (**High Sodium**)

Potassium: 339 mg
Calcium: 14 mg

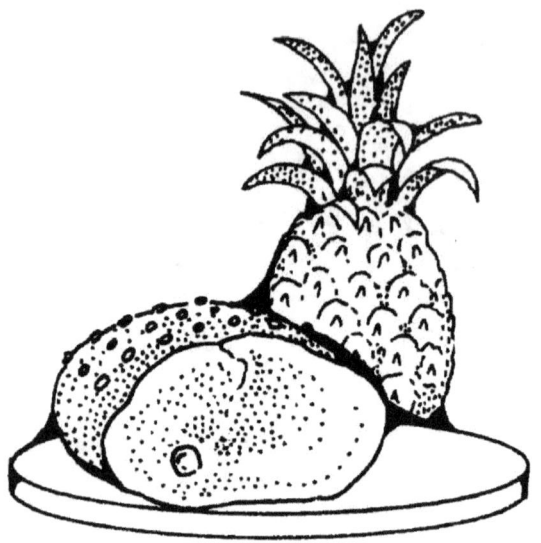

72

TURKEY STROGANOFF

4 cups cooked skinless turkey breast 1 tablespoon tomato paste

2 tablespoons margarine 1 teaspoon Worcestershire sauce

2 cups fresh sliced mushrooms 3 tablespoons cooking sherry

1 thinly-sliced onion ¾ cup low-fat sour cream

2 tablespoons flour

2 cups hot turkey or chicken broth, low-sodium, low-fat

Cut the cooked turkey into narrow strips and set aside. Melt one tablespoon of the margarine in a large skillet. Add the sliced mushrooms and onions; cook until tender and lightly browned. Remove the mushrooms and onions and put them in a bowl. Don't wash the pan. Melt the remaining one tablespoon margarine in the pan; add flour and stir until the flour is slightly browned. Add hot broth to the flour mixture, stirring constantly to form a smooth sauce. Add the tomato paste, Worcestershire sauce and sherry, stirring constantly. Simmer for 10 minutes. Add the turkey, mushrooms and onions to the pan and simmer for 10 minutes. Add the sour cream and mix thoroughly. Serve immediately over cooked noodles. Makes 8 (3/4 cup) servings.

One serving (no noodles):

Calories: 196

Carbohydrate: 6 grams

Protein: 24 grams

Cholesterol: 69 mg

Fiber: 1 grams

Sodium: 123 mg

Fat: 7 grams

Potassium: 409 mg

Saturated Fat: 3 grams

Calcium: 44 mg

Exchanges: ½ carbohydrate, 3 lean meat

One serving, served over one cup noodles:

Calories: 409

Cholesterol: 121 mg

Carbohydrate: 46 grams

Fiber: 3 grams

Protein: 32 grams

Sodium: 134 mg

Fat: 9 grams

Potassium: 454 mg

Saturated Fat: 3 grams

Calcium: 63 mg

Exchanges: 3 carbohydrates, 3 lean meat

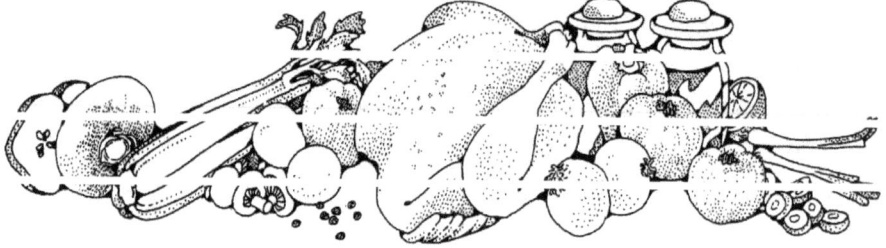

73

VEGETABLE LINGUINE

1 ¼ cup chopped onion
low-sodium tomato sauce
½ cup chopped celery
½ cup chopped green pepper
crushed red pepper flakes
2 minced garlic cloves
oregano
1 tablespoon olive oil
pepper
1 tablespoon dried basil
1 16-ounce can tomatoes

1 15-ounce can

2 teaspoons sugar
¼ teaspoon

½ teaspoon

1/8 teaspoon black

8 ounces Linguine

In a large sauce pan, sauté onion, celery, green pepper and garlic in olive oil until the vegetables are tender. Add remaining ingredients, except the linguine. Heat and simmer sauce for 30-40 minutes. Cook the linguine according to the package directions. Drain. Spoon the sauce over the cooked linguine. Serve immediately. Makes 6 servings.

One serving:
Calories: 233
Carbohydrate: 45 grams
Protein: 8 grams
Fat: 4 grams
Saturated Fat: 1 gram
Cholesterol: 0 mg
Fiber: 4 grams
Sodium: 161 mg
Potassium: 608 mg
Calcium: 68 mg
Exchanges: 2½ carbohydrates, 1 vegetable, ½ fat

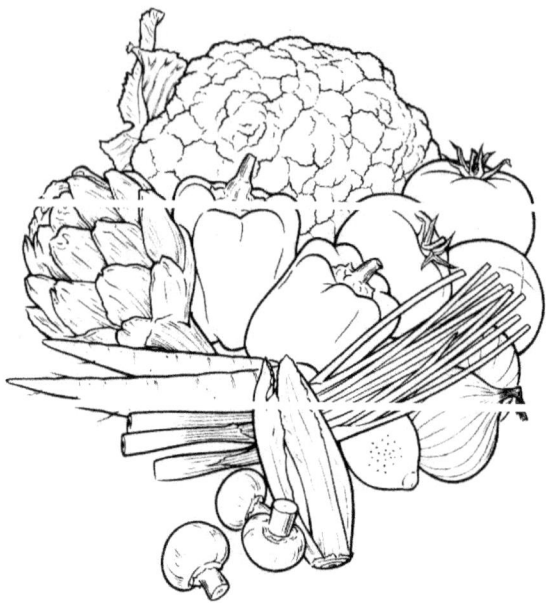

74

VEGETABLE LASAGNA

9 cooked lasagna noodles
2 cups sliced fresh mushrooms
1 cup chopped onion
1 tablespoon cooking oil
1 6-ounce can low-sodium tomato paste
1 15-ounce can low-sodium tomato sauce

1 teaspoon dried oregano
1 teaspoon dried basil
2 cups low-fat cottage cheese
1 cup shredded low-fat Monterey Jack Cheese
1 10-ounce package frozen, chopped spinach, thawed and well drained.

In a sauce pan, cook mushrooms and onion in oil until tender. Stir in tomato sauce, tomato paste, oregano and basil. In a mixing bowl, stir together cottage cheese and ½ cup of Monterey jack cheese. Oil a 3-quart rectangular baking dish. In the baking dish, layer three noodles, one-third of the cottage cheese mixture, one-third of the spinach, one-third of the tomato mixture. Repeat layers twice. Sprinkle with remaining Monterey Jack cheese. Bake, uncovered, at 375º for 30 minutes or until heated through. Let stand 10 minutes before serving. Makes 8 servings.

One serving:

Calories: 253
Carbohydrate: 32 grams
Protein: 17 grams
Fat: 8 grams
Saturated Fat: 3 grams
Cholesterol: 15 mg
Fiber: 4 grams
Sodium: 364 mg
Potassium: 686 mg
Calcium: 223 mg
Exchanges: 2 carbohydrates, ½ fat, 1½ lean meat

OVEN FRIED CHICKEN

6 skinless chicken breasts,
  (4 ounces each)
½ cup flour
1 teaspoon oil

½ teaspoon paprika
½ teaspoon garlic salt
¼ teaspoon black pepper

Preheat oven to 325º. Oil a 9x12-inch pan. Combine chicken, flour, paprika, garlic salt and pepper in a plastic bag. Shake. Place chicken on the oiled pan and bake for 25-35 minutes or until browned. Makes 6 servings.

One serving:

Calories: 188
Carbohydrate: 8 grams
Protein: 28 grams
Fat: 4 grams
Saturated Fat: 1 gram

Cholesterol: 73 mg
Fiber: 1 gram
Sodium: 153 mg
Potassium: 238 mg
Calcium: 15 mg

Exchanges: ½ carbohydrate, 4 very-lean meat

75

MARINATED STEAK

1 pound trimmed lean round steak
1 large sliced onion
½ cup low-sodium beef broth
2 tablespoons Worcestershire sauce

1 bay leaf
¼ teaspoon crushed red pepper
1/8 teaspoon allspice

Combine all ingredients in a large plastic bag. Seal and marinate in the refrigerator for at least 8 hours, turning occasionally. Remove steak from bag, reserving onion and marinade. Placed steak on rack of a broiler pan coated with non-stick cooking spray. Broil 7-8 minutes on each side or to desired degree of doneness. Set steak aside and keep warm. Coat a non -stick skillet with non-stick cooking spray, add onion and sauté over medium-high heat until tender. Add reserved marinade; cover and bring onion mixture to a boil, then reduce heat and simmer for 5 minutes. Remove and discard bay leaf. Transfer steak to a platter and spoon onion mixture over steak. Makes 4 servings.

One serving:

Calories: 182
Carbohydrate: 6 grams
Protein: 28 grams
Fat: 5 grams
Saturated Fat: 2 grams
Exchanges: 4 very-lean meat, 1 vegetable

Cholesterol: 71 mg
Fiber: 1 gram
Sodium: 150 mg
Potassium: 545 mg
Calcium: 25 mg

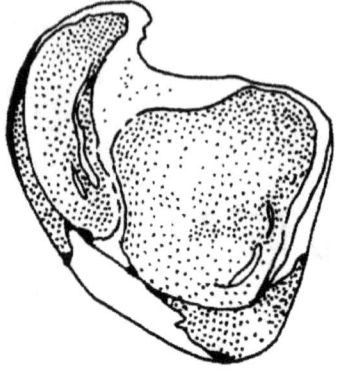

76

GRILLED LEMON CHICKEN

1/3 cup lemon juice

¼ cup water

½ teaspoon garlic powder

¼ teaspoon onion powder

1 teaspoon dried parsley

¼ teaspoon salt

4 small skinless chicken breasts (4 ounces each)

Mix all ingredients together except for the chicken breasts. Pour mixture over chicken. Let chicken marinate in the refrigerator for 2 hours or overnight. Grill over a slow charcoal or gas grill on low. Turn and marinate occasionally until done. Put reserved marinade into a saucepan and bring to a boil; serve on the side as a sauce.

One serving:

Calories: 148
Carbohydrate: 2 grams
Protein: 27 grams
Fat: 3 grams
Saturated Fat: 1 gram
Exchanges: 4 very-lean meat

Cholesterol: 73 mg
Fiber: trace
Sodium: 201 mg
Potassium: 248 mg
Calcium: 16 mg

GRILLED CHICKEN SALAD WITH RASPBERRY VINAIGRETTE

4 small skinless, boneless chicken breasts (about 4 ounces each)
¼ cup raspberry flavored vinegar   ¼ teaspoon sugar
½ teaspoon dried basil   ¼ teaspoon salt
¼ teaspoon garlic powder   8 cups salad greens
1 tablespoon olive oil

Grill chicken breasts on low, turning over until done. Combine the rest of the ingredients (except the salad greens) in a jar. Cover tightly and shake vigorously. Pour vinegar mixture over salad greens and toss gently. Divide salad greens on four plates. Cut each chicken breast into slices and arrange on top of greens. Serve immediately. Makes 4 servings.

One serving:

Calories: 192   Cholesterol: 73 mg
Carbohydrate: 4 grams   Fiber: 1 gram
Protein: 28 grams   Sodium: 207 mg
Fat: 7 grams   Potassium: 494 mg
Saturated Fat: 1 gram   Calcium: 48 mg
Exchanges: 1 vegetable, ½ fat, 4 very-lean meat

77

SWEET-AND-SOUR CHICKEN

1 pound skinless, boneless chicken breast, cut into 1-inch pieces

1 tablespoon cooking oil

1 cup chopped green pepper

1 cup carrots, sliced like coins

½ cup chopped onion

1 minced garlic clove

1 cup low-sodium chicken broth

1 tablespoon cornstarch

2 tablespoons brown sugar

2 tablespoons cooking sherry

½ teaspoon ground ginger

1 8-ounce can unsweetened pineapple chunks, drained

5 cups hot cooked rice

1 tablespoon low-sodium soy sauce

Heat oil in a large non-stick skillet over medium-high heat. Add chicken and stir-fry for five minutes or until chicken is browned. Add green pepper, carrot, onion and garlic. Stir-fry for 2 minutes. Combine broth, soy sauce, cornstarch, brown sugar, sherry and ginger; stir well. Add broth mixture and pineapple to skillet; bring to a boil and cook for one minute or until mixture is thickened and bubbly, stirring constantly. Serve over rice. Makes 8 servings.

One serving:

Calories: 307

Cholesterol: 36 mg

Carbohydrate: 48 grams

Fiber: 2 grams

Protein: 18 grams

Sodium: 185 mg

Fat: 4 grams

Potassium: 314 mg

Saturated Fat: 1 gram

Calcium: 37 mg

Exchanges: 3 carbohydrates, 1 lean meat

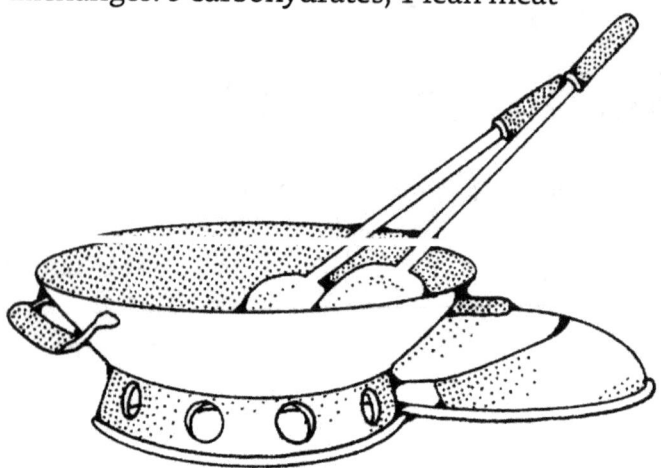

78

SPICY RED SNAPPER

1 pound fresh or frozen red snapper
2 tablespoons lime juice
ground ginger
½ teaspoon paprika
pepper

¼ teaspoon salt
¼ teaspoon
ground ginger

¼ teaspoon black

Rinse fish and pat dry with paper towels. Cut fish into 4 servings. Brush lime juice on top of fish. In a small bowl, combine paprika, salt, ginger and black pepper; rub onto fish. Arrange fish in a baking pan. Bake, uncovered, at 450º degrees for 10-15 minutes or until fish flakes easily when tested with a fork. Makes 4 servings.

One serving:
Calories: 112
Carbohydrate: 1 gram
Protein: 22 grams
Fat: 2 grams
Saturated Fat: 1 gram
Exchanges: 3 very-lean meat

Cholesterol: 40 mg
Fiber: trace
Sodium: 183 mg
Potassium: 460 mg
Calcium: 36 mg

LEMON BAKED SHRIMP

1 pound peeled, deveined shrimp

1/3 cup dry bread crumbs

1 teaspoon dried parsley

½ teaspoon grated lemon rind

1/8 teaspoon salt

2 minced garlic cloves

2 tablespoons fresh lemon juice

1 teaspoon olive oil

Coat 4 individual baking dishes with non -stick cooking spray. Divide shrimp between the dishes; set aside. Combine the bread crumbs, parsley, lemon rind, salt and garlic in a bowl; stir in lemon juice and olive oil. Sprinkle bread crumbs over the shrimp. Bake at 400º for 15 minutes or until shrimp are done and the bread crumb mixture is lightly browned. Makes 4 servings.

One serving:

Calories: 109

Carbohydrate: 7 grams

Protein: 14 grams

Fat: 2 grams

Saturated Fat: trace

Cholesterol: 121 mg

Fiber: 1 gram

Sodium: 278 mg

Potassium: 151 mg

Calcium: 48 mg

Exchanges: ½ carbohydrate, ½ fat, 1 ½ very -lean meat

79

184

SLOPPY JOES

1 pound extra-lean ground beef ¼ teaspoon
dry mustard
¼ cup tomato juice 2
tablespoons ketchup
¼ cup ground onion ½
teaspoon salt
1 tablespoon prepared mustard

Brown ground beef and onions. Drain off fat. Add remaining ingredients. Simmer for 20-30 minutes. Serve on a bun. Makes 6 servings.

One serving on a bun:

Calories: 250
Carbohydrate: 24 grams
Protein: 16 grams
Sodium)
Fat: 9 grams
Saturated Fat: 3 grams

Cholesterol: 42 mg
Fiber: 1 gram
Sodium: 451 mg (**High**

Potassium: 263 mg
Calcium: 71 mg

Exchanges: 1½ carbohydrates, 2 medium-fat meat

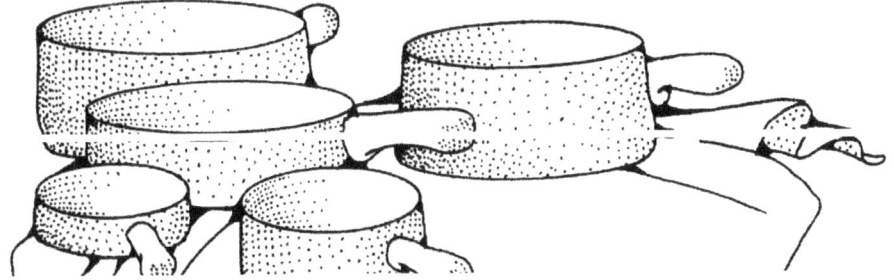

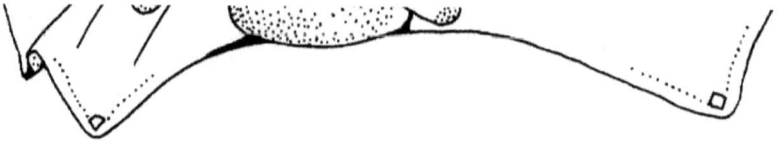

80

DESSERTS

APPLE CRUNCH

6 cups thinly sliced cooking apples
¼ cup brown sugar powder
½ teaspoon cinnamon
½ cup sugar margarine

1 ½ cups flour
1 teaspoon baking

1 egg, beaten
½ cup melted

Place apples in a 13x9-inch pan. Combine brown sugar and cinnamon; sprinkle over apples. Mix sugar, flour and baking powder. Work egg into flour mixture with a fork. Sprinkle flour mixture over apples. Drizzle melted margarine over all. Bake at 325º approximately 45 minutes or until crunch top is golden. Makes 18 servings.

One serving:

Calories: 148
Carbohydrate: 24 grams
Protein: 2 grams
Fat: 6 grams
Saturated Fat: 1 gram
Exchanges: 1 ½ carbohydrates, 1 fat, 1 fruit

Cholesterol: 10 mg
Fiber: 1 gram
Sodium: 74 mg
Potassium: 65 mg
Calcium: 24 mg

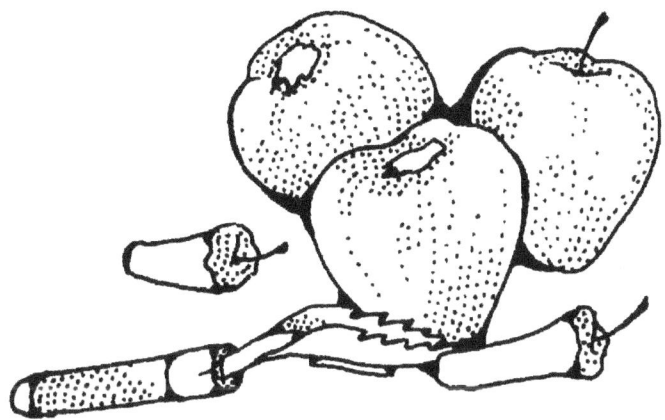

81

PEACH CRUNCH

4 cups fresh or drained, canned peaches (packed in juice)

¼ cup sugar

2 tablespoons flour

½ teaspoon cinnamon

1 teaspoon vanilla

1 cup oatmeal

½ cup flour

1 teaspoon cinnamon

4 tablespoons diet margarine

In a bowl, add peaches, sugar, flour, 2 tablespoons flour, ½ teaspoon cinnamon and vanilla. Mix well and set aside. In a separate bowl, combine oatmeal, ½ cup flour and one teaspoon cinnamon. Cut in diet margarine until mixture is crumbly in texture. Place the peach mixture in bottom of an 8x8-inch pan. Sprinkle the oatmeal mixture over the peaches. Bake at 350º for 30-40 minutes, or until the crust is golden brown. Makes 8 servings.

One serving:

Calories: 166

Carbohydrate: 30 grams

Protein: 3 grams

Fat: 4 grams

Saturated Fat: 1 gram

Exchanges: 2 carbohydrates, ½ fat

Cholesterol: 0 mg

Fiber: 3 grams

Sodium: 56 mg

Potassium: 217 mg

Calcium: 17 mg

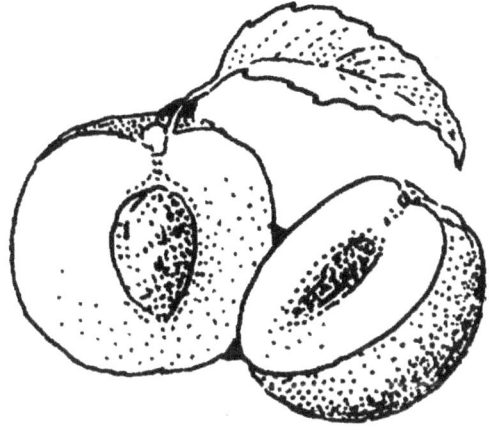

82

LEMON CHERRY CHEESECAKE

1 whole graham cracker, crushed

1 package sugar-free lemon gelatin

2/3 cup boiling water

1 cup low-fat cottage cheese

8 ounces fat-free cream cheese

2 cups low-fat whipped topping

1 cup low-sugar cherry pie filling

Spray an 8-inch spring form pan or a 9-inch pie plate lightly with non-stick cooking spray. Sprinkle bottom with graham cracker crumbs. Dissolve gelatin in boiling water; pour into blender. Add cottage cheese and fat-free cream cheese. Cover and blend at medium speed, scraping down sides, until smooth. Pour into a large bowl and gently stir in whipped topping. Pour into pan. Chill until set (about 4 hours). When ready to serve, top cheesecake with cherry pie filling. Makes 8 servings.

One serving:

Calories: 94

Carbohydrate: 12 grams

Protein: 8 grams

Fat: 2 grams

Saturated Fat: 1 gram

Cholesterol: 26 mg

Fiber: trace

Sodium: 300 mg

Potassium: 92 mg

Calcium: 43 mg

Exchanges: 1 carbohydrate, 1/2 very-lean meat

STRAWBERRIES AND CREAM

2 cups skim milk ½ teaspoon almond extract
¼ cup sugar 3 cups strawberries
2 tablespoons cornstarch

Combine milk, sugar and cornstarch in a saucepan. Cook over medium heat, stirring constantly, until mixture comes to a boil. Stir in almond extract. Cover and chill thoroughly. Place ½ cup of strawberries in each of 6 individual dessert dishes. Pour cream mixture over each serving. Makes 6 servings.

One serving:

Calories: 86
Carbohydrate: 18 grams
Protein: 3 grams
Fat: 1 gram
Saturated Fat: trace
Exchanges: 1 carbohydrate

Cholesterol: 2 mg
Fiber: 1 gram
Sodium: 43 mg
Potassium: 274 mg
Calcium: 112 mg

83

PINEAPPLE-PISTACHIO MOUSSE

1 small package sugar-free pistachio instant pudding mix
1 8-ounce carton plain low-fat yogurt
1 8-ounce carton vanilla low-fat, sugar-free yogurt
1 8-ounce can unsweetened crushed pineapple, drained
1 cup low-fat whipped topping

Combine pudding mix, plain yogurt, vanilla yogurt and pineapple; stir well. Fold in whipped topping. Spoon into 6 individual dessert bowls. Chill. Makes 6 servings.

One serving:

Calories: 92
Carbohydrate: 16 grams
Protein: 3 grams
Fat: 3 grams
Saturated Fat: 2 grams
Exchanges: 1 carbohydrate, ½ fat

Cholesterol: 6 mg
Fiber: trace
Sodium: 181 mg
Potassium: 257 mg
Calcium: 104 mg

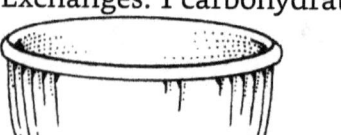

Baked Custard

2 cups skim milk

2 tablespoons sugar

2 teaspoons vanilla extract

¾ cup non-fat egg substitute

Mix milk, sugar, vanilla and egg substitute. Pour the custard mixture into four oven-proof custard dishes. Place the custard dishes in a deep pan; fill the pan with hot water up to the level of the custard. Bake in a preheated oven at 325º for 45-60 minutes. The custard is done when it is firm in the center. Serve warm or chilled. Makes 4 servings.

One serving:

Calories: 130

Carbohydrate: 21 grams

Protein: 8 grams

Fat: 2 grams

Saturated Fat: trace

Exchanges: 1 1/2 carbohydrates

Cholesterol: 19 mg

Fiber: 0 mg

Sodium: 106 mg

Potassium: 242 mg

Calcium: 155 mg

84

CHERRY CRISP

1 can low-sugar cherry pie filling
1/3 cup flour
1 cup oatmeal

¼ cup brown sugar
3 tablespoons margarine

Spread cherry pie filling in an 8x8- inch baking dish. Mix flour, oatmeal and brown sugar together. Cut margarine into oatmeal mixture. Crumble oatmeal mixture over the top of the cherries. Bake at 375º for 30 minutes. Makes 8 servings.

One serving:
Calories: 147
Carbohydrate: 25 grams
Protein: 2 grams
Fat: 5 grams
Saturated Fat: 1 gram
Exchanges: 1 1/2 carbohydrates, 1 fat

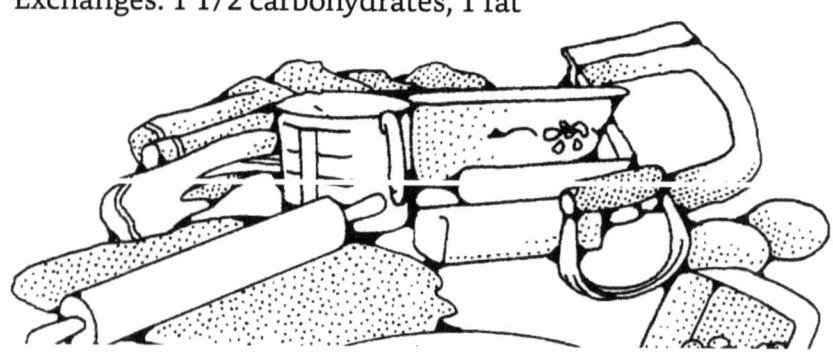

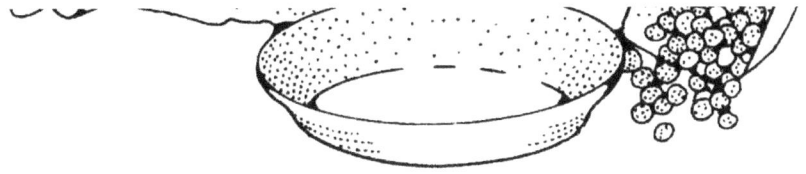

Cholesterol: 0 mg
Fiber: 2 grams
Sodium: 40 mg
Potassium: 97 mg
Calcium: 15 mg

85

WHOLE WHEAT CINNAMON SUGAR COOKIES

1 cup sugar

1 tablespoon lemon or orange peel

1 teaspoon baking powder

1 teaspoon vanilla extract

½ teaspoon salt

1 egg

½ teaspoon soda

2 cups whole wheat flour

½ teaspoon nutmeg

2 tablespoons sugar

½ cup softened margarine

½ teaspoon cinnamon

3 tablespoons milk

In a large bowl, combine sugar, baking powder, salt, soda, nutmeg, margarine, milk, lemon or orange peel, vanilla and egg. Blend well. Stir in flour. Cover and chill for 30-60 minutes. On a lightly floured surface, roll out dough to 1/8-inch thickness. Cut with floured cutters. Place on ungreased cookie sheets, two inches apart. Combine 2 tablespoons sugar and ½ teaspoon cinnamon; sprinkle over cookies. Bake at 375º for 8-10 minutes, or until lightly golden brown. Let stand one minute. Remove from cookie sheets and cool. Makes 36 cookies.

One cookie:

Calories: 72

Cholesterol: 5 mg

Carbohydrate: 11 grams
Protein: 1 grams
Fat: 3 grams
Saturated Fat: 1 gram
Exchanges: 1 carbohydrate, ½ fat

Fiber: 1 gram
Sodium: 85 mg
Potassium: 33 mg
Calcium: 14 mg

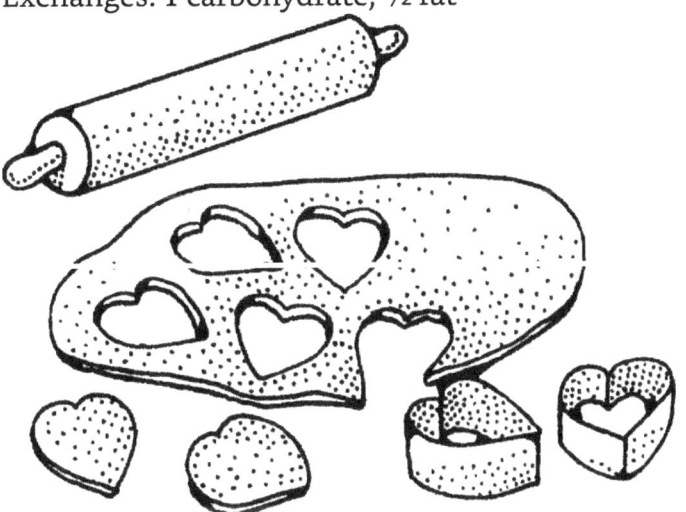

86

ANGEL FOOD CAKE

1 cup cake flour, sifted
1 teaspoon cream of tartar ¼ cup sugar twin

1 cup egg whites (8-10 eggs) ½ teaspoon vanilla extract

Sift 1/8 cup sugar twin and flour together four times. Beat egg whites and cream of tartar until foamy. Add remaining sugar twin a little at a time, beating in well. Add vanilla and beat until very stiff. Fold flour into egg white and sugar mixture, small amounts at a time. Pour into 10-inch ungreased tube pan. Cut through with a spatula to remove air bubbles. Bake at 275º for 30 minutes, then raise the heat to 300º and bake until done. Invert pan for one hour before removing from pan. Makes 12 servings.

One serving:

Calories: 44

Carbohydrate: 7 grams

Protein: 3 grams

Fat: trace

Saturated Fat: trace

Exchanges: ½ carbohydrate

Cholesterol: 0 mg

Fiber: trace

Sodium: 44 mg

Potassium: 91 mg

Calcium: 7 mg

PINEAPPLE CAKE

2 cups flour
1 ¼ cups sugar
2 eggs
pineapple
1 teaspoon baking soda

1 teaspoon vanilla
¼ teaspoon salt
1 16-ounce can crushed

in its own juice

Mix all ingredients together. Pour into a greased and floured 9x13-inch pan. Bake at 325º for 35-40 minutes. Makes 24 servings.

One serving:

Calories: 97
Carbohydrate: 22 grams
Protein: 2 grams
Fat: 1 gram
Saturated Fat: trace
Exchanges: 1 1/2 carbohydrates

Cholesterol: 16 mg
Fiber: 1 gram
Sodium: 80 mg
Potassium: 41 mg
Calcium: trace

87

PINEAPPLE PUMPKIN PIE

Filling:

2 envelopes unflavored gelatin

3 tablespoons cool water

1 cup skim milk

1/4 cup boiling water

1 ½ teaspoons cinnamon

1 16-ounce can pumpkin

¼ teaspoon ginger

1 8-ounce can crushed pineapple in juice

1/8 teaspoon ground cloves

2 tablespoons sugar

2 teaspoons vanilla

Crust:

1 cup graham cracker crumbs

2 tablespoons melted margarine

2 tablespoons sugar

Mix all of the crust ingredients together and pat into a 9-inch pie pan. Soften the gelatin in cool water for 5 minutes. Add boiling water and stir until the gelatin is completely dissolved. Put the gelatin mixture and all the other filling ingredients in a blender and blend until smooth and frothy. Allow the mixture to stand until slightly thickened before pouring into the graham cracker crust. Chill for at least 3 hours before serving. Makes 8 servings.

One serving:

Calories: 172

Carbohydrate: 30 grams

Protein: 5 grams

Cholesterol: trace

Fiber: 3 grams

Sodium: 138 mg

Fat: 5 grams
Saturated Fat: 1 gram
Exchanges: 2 carbohydrates, 1 fat

Potassium: 268 mg
Calcium: 71 mg

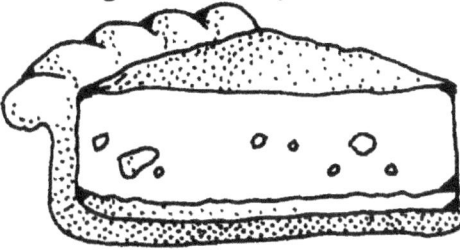

88

MISCELLANEOUS

FRESH SALSA

4 large fresh tomatoes, chopped
juice
1 4-ounce can green chilies
1 medium onion, chopped
ground pepper
1 fresh jalapeno, chopped
½ teaspoon cumin

2 teaspoons lime

1 teaspoon cilantro
½ teaspoon

¼ teaspoon salt

Mix all ingredients together and chill. Makes approximately four cups.

¼ cup serving:

Calories: 15
Carbohydrate: 4 grams
Protein: 1 gram
Fat: trace
Saturated Fat: trace
Exchanges: One Serving Free

Cholesterol: 0 mg
Fiber: 1 gram
Sodium: 121 mg
Potassium: 128 mg
Calcium: 5 mg

BLACK BEAN SALSA

1 15-ounce can black beans, rinsed and drained
1 cup chopped tomatoes 1 4-ounce can green chilies, drained
½ cup low-sodium corn, drained 1 teaspoon lime juice
½ cup chopped onion 1/8 teaspoon black pepper
1 minced garlic clove

Combine all ingredients and let stand in the refrigerator for at least one hour. Makes 3 cups.

¼ cup serving:

Calories: 89
Carbohydrate: 17 grams
Protein: 5 grams
Fat: 1 gram
Saturated Fat: trace

Cholesterol: 0 mg
Fiber: 5 grams
Sodium: 276 mg
Potassium: 292 mg
Calcium: 18 mg

89

Exchanges: 1 carbohydrate

MILD GARLIC MARINADE

2 tablespoons cooking oil
3 tablespoons wine vinegar
pepper
1/3 cup tomato juice chopped
¼ teaspoon salt

1 teaspoon paprika
½ teaspoon black

2 garlic cloves,

Mix all ingredients together. Cover desired meat in marinade and chill in the refrigerator for at least one hour. Grill, roast, broil or bake meat as desired. Makes ¾ cup marinade.

One tablespoon:

Calories: 23
Carbohydrate: 1 gram
Protein: trace
Fat: 3 grams
Saturated Fat: trace
Exchanges: ½ fat

Cholesterol: 0 mg
Fiber: trace
Sodium: 25 mg
Potassium: 26 mg
Calcium: 3 mg

RANCH STYLE DRESSING MIX

1 cup non-fat dry milk powder
4 teaspoons dried basil
2 tablespoons minced dried onion

2 teaspoons dry mustard

1 teaspoon garlic powder
½ teaspoon salt

Combine all ingredients in a bowl. Stir well. Store in an airtight container. To use: combine 1/4 cup of mix with 1/4 cup water. Blend into 1 cup non-fat plain yogurt. Shake well before serving. One serving equals 2 tablespoons.

One serving (prepared):

Calories: 25
Carbohydrate: 4 grams
Protein: 2 grams
Fat: trace
Saturated Fat: trace
Exchanges: ¼ carbohydrate

Cholesterol: 1 mg
Fiber: trace
Sodium: 60 mg
Potassium: 117 mg
Calcium: 87 mg

90

DIABETES RESOURCES

Nebraska Diabetes Prevention & Control Program
http://www.hhs.state.ne.us/dpc/ndcp.htm

This home page tells you about the Nebraska Department of Health & Human Services, Diabetes Prevention & Control Program. The quarterly newsletter, a list of materials, and links to other diabetes home pages are available on this site.

Division of Diabetes Translation at the Centers for Disease Prevention and Control (CDC)
http://www.cdc.gov/diabetes

This site tells you about the CDC's Division of Diabetes Translation and its current projects to reduce the burden of diabetes. This site links to information about many of the State-based Diabetes Control Programs. There is a frequently asked questions section and links to other diabetes home pages.

National Institute of Diabetes and Digestive and Kidney Diseases (NIDDK) Home Page
http://www.niddk.nih.gov/

This site provides consumer health information on disorders covered by NIDDK. It covers research, recent news releases and links to other U.S. Government health information sources. This home page provides National Diabetes Clearinghouse (NDIC) publications for health professionals and patients.

The National Eye Institute (NEI)
http://www.nei.nigh.gov/

This site provides information on eye health and eye diseases, including information about eye diseases prevalent to people with diabetes such as: retinopathy, glaucoma, and cataracts. This home page offers press releases about study findings and information on clinical studies.

National Diabetes Education Program
http://ndep.nih.gov and http://www.betterdiabetescare.org
These sites provide information and resources on the National Diabetes Education Program that is co-sponsored by the Centers for Disease Prevention and Control and the National Institutes of Health.

Centers for Medicare and Medicaid Services
http://cms.hhs.gov or http://www.medicare.gov
These sites provide information about diabetes and Medicare

benefits. **The National Center for Health Statistics (NCHS)**
http://www.cdc.gov/nchs

This home page for NCHS provides information about publications, electronic products, and the Center's activities.

Indian Health Service (I H S)
http://www.his.gov/
This home page offers several links to American Indian health information as well as a link
for health care providers and to
I H S publications.

91

National Institute of Dental Research (NIDR) http://www.nidr.nih.gov
This site includes information about dental complications of diabetes. NIDR's publications cover diabetes and periodontal disease, and dental tips for people with diabetes.

American Association of Diabetes Educators
http://www.diabeteseducator.org
This home page lists information on the organization, professional education and legislation.
Publications available are listed. Links are available to other diabetes information sources.

American Diabetes Association (ADA)
http://www.diabetes.org
This site provides information on membership, what's new in diabetes and access to ADA's information center. The site links to most ADA State Affiliate web sites.

Nebraska Dietetic Association http://www.eatrightnebraska.org

American Dietetic Association (ADA)
http://www.eatright.org
This home page contains information about ADA and the National Center for Dietetics (NCND). It includes a list of nutrition resources, fact sheets, and hot topics.

Juvenile Diabetes Research Foundation
http://www.jdrf.org
This home page provides information about JDRF, research efforts and publications available. Membership information is included as well as chapter information.

Juvenile Diabetes Research Foundation/Lincoln Chapter
http://www.jdrforg/lincoln

Juvenile Diabetes Research Foundation
Omaha/Council Bluffs Chapter
http://www.jdrf.org/chapters/NE/Omaha-Council-Bluffs

American Association of Clinical Endocrinologists (AACE)
http://www.aace.com
This site features a Members Area, which includes membership information, discussion groups and legislative information. The Public Area includes a definition of AACE, clinical guidelines and a guide to related endocrinology sites.

International Diabetic Athletes Association (IDAA) http://diabetes-exercise.org/

This site provides information on how to become a member, meeting and support group information, and how to obtain a mail order catalog of IDAA's materials.

International Diabetes Federation (IDF)

http://www.idf.org

This site provides information on diabetes. Membership and contact information is listed.

Preview Federation publications. Discover diabetes happenings around the world.

92

Joslin Diabetes Center
http://www.joslin.harvard.edu/

This site describes the Joslin Diabetes Center, and provides the Center's location, satellite sites and affiliated centers. The site lists Joslin publications, research studies and frequently asked questions about diabetes.

Diabetes Net
http://www.diabetesnet.com

This web site hosts a Diabetes Mall. Information on insulin therapy, diabetes complications, books, cookbooks, and links to other diabetes sites are provided. The Mall advertises products that are usually created and sold by people with diabetes.

Health Disparities Collaboratives
http://www.healthdisparities.net

This site provides information and resources used in a national effort to improve health outcomes for all medically underserved people with chronic disease.

Barbara Davis Center for Childhood Diabetes http://www.barbaradaviscenter.org

This site provides information about Type I diabetes, research and publications. It also describes the Barbara Davis Center.

Children's Diabetes Foundation
http://www.childrensdiabetesfdn.org

This site provides information on education, publications, recipes and events geared towards children with diabetes.

93

Diabetes Internet Resources

Nebraska Diabetes Prevention & Control Program
http://www.dhhs.ne.gov/dpc/ndcp.htm

CDC Division of Diabetes Translation
http://www.cdc.gov/diabetes

Administration on Aging
http://www.aoa.gov

American Association of Diabetes Educators (AADE)
http://www.diabeteseducator.org

American Diabetes Association (ADA)
http://www.diabetes.org

American Dietetic Association (ADA)
http://www.eatright.org

American Heart Association
http://www.americanheart.org

CDC Division of Nutrition and Physical Activity
http://www.cdc.gov/nccdphp/dnpa

Centers for Medicare and Medicaid Services
http://cms.hhs.gov **or** http://www.medicare.gov

CIMRO of Nebraska
http://cimronebraska.org

U.S. HHSS, Department of Veterans Affairs
http://www.va.gov/health/diabetes

U.S. HHSS, Health Resources and Services Administration http://www.hrsa.gov

U.S. HHSS, Indian Health Service (IHS)
http://www.ihs.gov/

International Diabetes Exercise & Sports Association (DESA)
http://www.diabetes-exercise.org

International Diabetes Federation (IDF)
http://www.idf.org

Joslin Diabetes Center
http://www.joslin.harvard.edu/

Juvenile Diabetes Research Foundation International (JDRF)
http://www.jdrf.org

94

The National Center for Health Statistics (NCHS) http://www.cdc.gov/nchs **National Certification Board for Diabetes Educators** http://www.ncbde.org **National Diabetes Education Program (NDEP)**

http://ndep.nih.gov
http://www.cdc.gov/team-ndep
http://betterdiabetescare.nih.gov
http://www.YourDiabetesInfo.org
http://www.diabetesinformation.org
http://www.diabetesinformacion.org (for
   Spanish-language materials)

The National Eye Institute
http://www.nei.nih.gov

National Health Information Center
http://www.health.gov/nhic

National Institute of Dental & Cranofacial Research (NIDCR)
http://www.nidcr.nih.gov

National Institute of Diabetes and Digestive and Kidney Diseases (NIDDK) Diabetes Home Page www2.niddk.nih.gov

National Diabetes Information Clearing House (NDIC) http://www.diabetes.niddk.nih.gov/

National Library Service for the Blind and Physically Handicapped (NLS) http://www.loc.gov/nls

Nebraska Library Commission
http://www.nlc.state.ne.us

The National Women's Health Information Center http://www.womenshealth.gov

U.S. Food and Drug Administration
http://www.fda.gov
FDA Diabetes Site http://www.fda.gov/diabetes

U.S. HHSS, Office of Minority Health
http://www.omhrc.gov

Nebraska Diabetes Prevention & Control Program
301 Centennial Mall South
P.O. Box 95026
Lincoln, NE 68509-5026
1-800-745-9311
E-mail: dhhs.diabetes@nebraska.gov

95

INDEX

Bean Dip, 27	Cabbage - Sweet & Sour, 63
Bean (Black) Salsa, 91	Cafe Au Lait (Cinnamon), 34
Beans (Red) & Rice, 65	Cake - Angel Food, 89
Beef Burgundy, 73	Cake - Pineapple, 89
Beverages, 29-34	Carrot & Tuna Salad, 50
Blueberry Smoothie, 31	Carrot Raisin Salad, 44
Champagne Imposter, 32	Casserole - Green Bean, 61
Cinnamon Cafe Au Lait, 34	Casserole - Green Bean & Rice, 63
Cranberry Punch, 32	Casserole - Northlands Wild Rice, 67
Cran-Raspberry Tea, 29	Cauliflower & Broccoli Salad, 48
Hot Cocoa, 33	Celery-Cranberry Mold, 45
Hot Spiced Tomato Juice, 33	Champagne Imposter, 32
Lime Cooler, 30	Cheese Potato Fries - Microwaved, 62
Pineapple Smoothie, 31	Cheesecake - Lemon Cherry, 85
Special Tea, 29	Cherry Crisp, 87
Simmered Cider, 30	Cherry Lemon Cheesecake, 85
Biscuits, 35	Chicken Cilantro, 69
Biscuits - Cinnamon-Raisin, 36	Chicken Enchiladas, 70
Black Bean Salsa, 91	Chicken - Grilled Lemon, 79
Blueberry Smoothie, 31	Chicken Noodle Soup (Homestyle), 56
Bolillos, 41	Chicken - Oven Fried, 77
Bread - Cranberry, 40	Chicken Salad, 51

Bread Stuffing, 6		
	96	

Chicken Salad - Grilled w/Raspberry Vinaigrette, 79

Apple Salad, 43
Apricot Salad, 43
Broccoli & Bean Salad, 48
Broccoli & Cauliflower Salad, 48
Broccoli & Shrimp Salad, 51
Buttermilk Salad Dressing, 52

98

Carrot Raisin Salad, 44

Turkey Chili, 56

Bread Stuffing, 66
Festive Rice, 65
Garbanzo Bean & Tomato Sauce, 59
Green Been Casserole, 61
Green Bean &Rice Casserole, 63
Grilled Vegetables & Potatoes, 62
Italian-Mexican Vegetable Bake, 59
Microwaved Cheese Potato Fries, 62
Northlands Wild Rice Casserole, 67
Parmesan Basil Tomatoes, 60
Red Beans & Rice, 65
Rice , 64
Scalloped Corn, 60
Spanish Rice, 64
Sweet & Sour Cabbage, 63
Twice Baked Yams, 61
Wild Rice Casserole, 66
Vinaigrette/Raspberry-Grilled Chicken
    Salad, 79
Waldorf Salad, 44
Whole Wheat Cinnamon Sugar Cookies, 88
Wild Rice Casserole, 66
Wild Rice - Northlands Casserole, 67
Yams - Twice Baked, 61

99